DIAGNOSTIC PICTURE TESTS IN
PAEDIATRICS

Second edition

R.D.G. Milner
MA, MD, PhD, ScD, FRCP

Professor and Head, Department of Paediatrics
University of Sheffield, England

S.M. Herber
MB, BCh, MRCP

Lecturer, Department of Paediatrics
University of Sheffield, England

Glaxo

Copyright © R.D.G. Milner & S.M. Herber, 1990
Published by Wolfe Medical Publications Ltd, 1990
Printed by Grafos, Arte Sobre Papel, Barcelona, Spain
ISBN 0 7234 1599 4

A CIP catalogue record for this book is available from the British Library.

For a full list of Wolfe Medical Atlases, plus forthcoming titles and details of our surgical, dental and veterinary Atlases, please write to Wolfe Medical Publications Limited, Brook House, 2–16 Torrington Place, London WC1E 7LT England.

Preface

In common with all clinical specialities, correct diagnosis in paediatrics is largely dependent upon careful history and examination but the possibilities for 'spot' diagnosis do exist. In this second edition, approximately one-third of the questions and answers have been replaced, both to produce a wide range of self assessment exercises and to reflect changes in diagnosis (and diagnostic tools) since the first edition was produced. We estimate that an undergraduate should be able to solve a third of the set questions, while the average postgraduate candidate is expected to answer a further third. It is hoped that the book as a whole will prove to be a stimulus to further reading for both undergraduates and postgraduates. The authors would like to thank their own examination candidates who served, unknowingly in many respects, as the moderators of some of the questions.

Acknowledgements

We wish to thank the Departments of Medical Illustration at the Northern General Hospital and Royal Hallamshire Hospital, Sheffield, for their assistance with photography and duplication. We are grateful to Mrs G Wilson for her patient typing of the text and we thank Dr R A Primhak for helpful discussion. The generous co-operation of the following colleagues who provided slides is appreciated:

Dr A W Boon

Mr J A S Dickson

Professor B I Duerden

Dr M B Duggan

Dr J M King

Dr R K Levick

Dr J S Lilleyman

Mr A E MacKinnon

Dr J E Oliver

Dr R G Pearse

Dr M Placzek

Dr D A Price

Dr B L Priestley

Dr R A Primhak

Dr M F Smith

Mr R Spicer

Professor L Spitz

Dr G M Steiner

Dr L S Taitz

Dr S Variend

Dr J K H Wales

Dr G Whincup

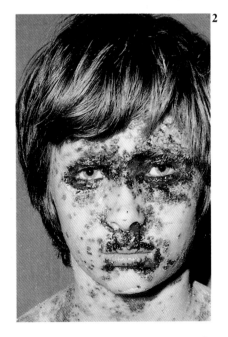

1 (a) List two abnormalities demonstrated in this cranial ultrasound examination of a preterm infant.

(b) What is the long term prognosis for normal development?

2 (a) What condition is demonstrated in this nine-year-old atopic boy?

(b) What is the treatment of choice?

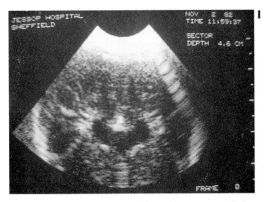

3

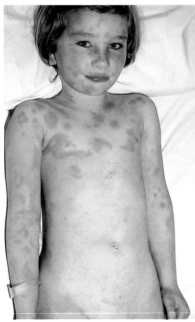

3 A boy was admitted to hospital the previous day with fever, malaise and this obvious skin rash.

(a) What is the name of the rash?

(b) What part of the body is characteristically avoided in this eruption?

(c) What is the treatment of choice?

4 This infant felt floppy when handled by the nurse. Name five possible causes of such floppiness.

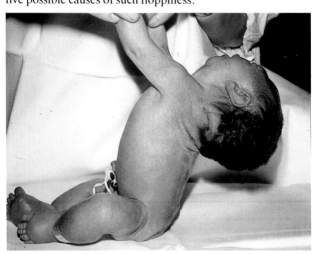

5 This radiograph shows contrast medium in the stomach during the course of a barium meal examination.

(a) What abnormality is shown?

(b) What is the commonest cause of this abnormality?

(c) What is the most likely clinical presentation?

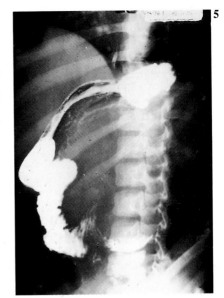

6 This is a slide of a six-year-old with cystic fibrosis.

(a) What is demonstrated?

(b) How can this be prevented?

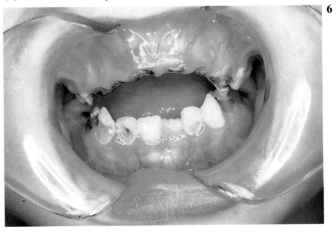

7

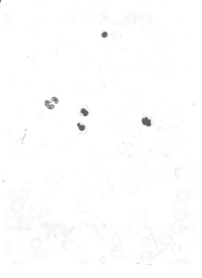

7 Describe four abnormalities shown in this peripheral blood film taken from a five-year-old West Indian boy.

8

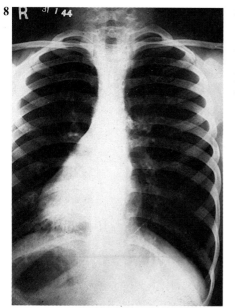

8 (a) What condition does this radiograph demonstrate?
(b) With what syndrome is this associated?
(c) Name two further pathological features of the syndrome.

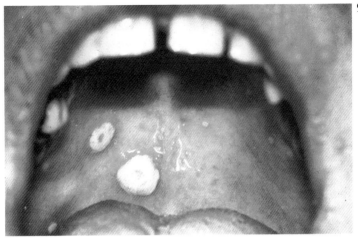

9 A nine-year-old boy was admitted to hospital, having been feverish and systemically unwell for two days. Physical examination was within normal limits except for the lesions shown here and four macules on the neck.
(a) What is the likely diagnosis?
(b) State three ways in which the diagnosis may be confirmed.

10 (a) What defect is demonstrated in this stillborn fetus?
(b) Before what intrauterine age must the defect of embryogenesis occur to produce this?

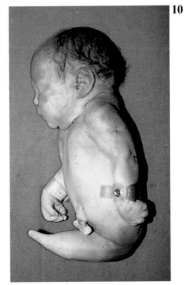

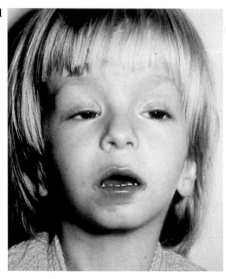

11 A child has a diagnostically characteristic facies.
(a) What condition does he have?
(b) Name three other characteristics of the condition.

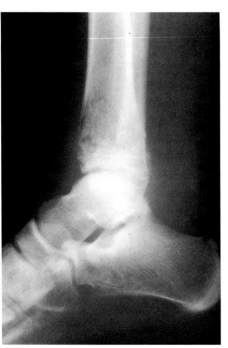

12 This eight-year-old presented acutely ill with a swollen ankle.
(a) What is the diagnosis?
(b) What treatment is required?
(c) Name four organisms that may cause this.

13 A stocky seven-year-old boy was referred to the hospital as an emergency by the Social Services Department. The family has been followed for several years because of poor home circumstances. His teacher and neighbours had complained that the boy had excessive bruising. On examination the bruises shown were the only abnormal findings. Investigations showed the platelet count to be normal, the prothrombin time and thrombin time were normal, but the bleeding time was 17 minutes. No history of drug ingestion could be elicited.

(a) What is the most likely diagnosis?

(b) Name two confirmatory tests.

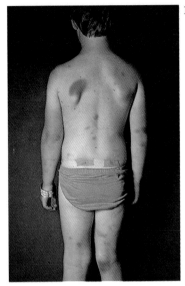

14 This is a slide of a three-year-old.

(a) What condition is demonstrated?

(b) Name two possible causes.

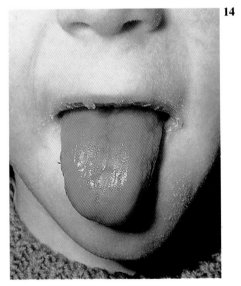

15

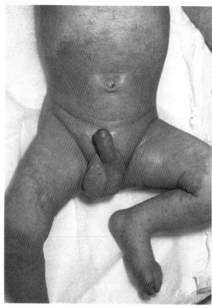

15 A mother presented at an infant welfare clinic with her three-month-old infant, complaining that he had a nappy rash.

(a) What is the cause of the nappy rash?

(b) Name two organisms which commonly cause superinfection.

(c) What other part of the body characteristically may be affected?

16 A three-year-old was brought to the Accident and Emergency Department because she refused to swallow and was drooling.

(a) What condition is demonstrated?

(b) What is responsible for the acute inflammation and ulceration of the throat?

(c) What treatment is available?

16

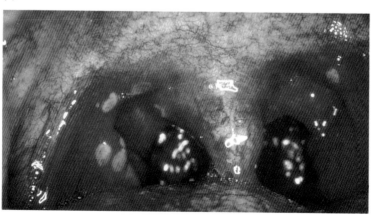

17 (a) What is striking about the body habitus of this 13-year-old?
(b) How might this be caused?

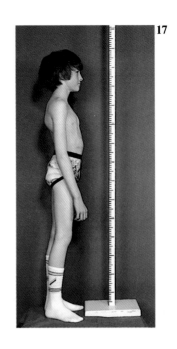

18 This is a radiograph of a healthy nine-year-old found to have a systolic murmur.
(a) Name two abnormalities present.
(b) What diagnosis do these suggest?
(c) What may the ECG show?

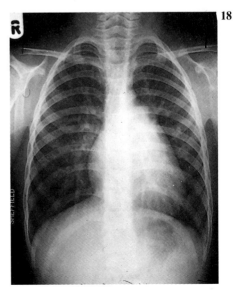

19

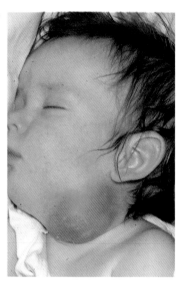

19 An 18-month-old infant with bilateral swelling of the neck was taken to his general practitioner, who diagnosed tonsillitis. Five days later he was brought to hospital with the swelling as shown. Examination of the mouth revealed pus at the opening of Stensen's duct.
(a) What condition is illustrated?
(b) In which common illness may this be a complication?
(c) What is the most common causative organism?

20

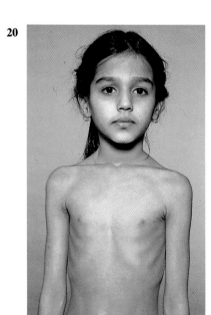

20 (a) What is the diagnosis in this six-year-old Asian girl who has a small chest?
(b) How is the condition inherited?

21 This is a child with the characteristic facies of a mucopolysaccharidosis. In the evaluation of such a patient, state three important features in the history and clinical examination that may help in differentiating between the Hunter and the Hurler syndromes.

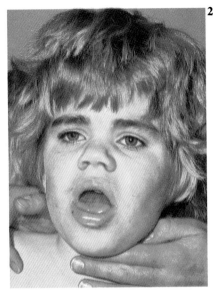

22 A baby was taken to the family doctor with a rash around the mouth. The lesions were swabbed but no organism could be cultured.
(a) What is the likely diagnosis?
(b) What is the explanation for the colour of the lesions?
(c) What treatment may be of benefit?

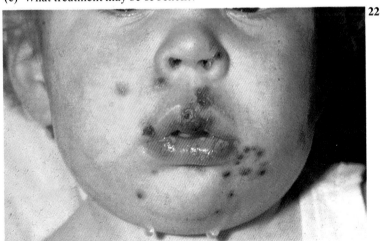

23 (a) What examination is being performed in this radiograph?
(b) What is demonstrated?

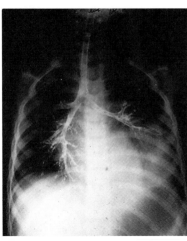

24 An eight-year-old girl presented with a five-month history of weight loss, abdominal pain and intermittent diarrhoea. Blood had been noticed in her stools on two occasions. She also complained of a sore mouth.
(a) What is the likely diagnosis?
(b) What abnormality is shown?
(c) What is the investigation of choice to help to prove the diagnosis?

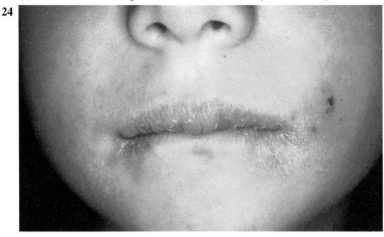

25 A diabetic girl complained of the shape of her thighs.
(a) What abnormality is illustrated?
(b) State two ways in which the condition may be treated.

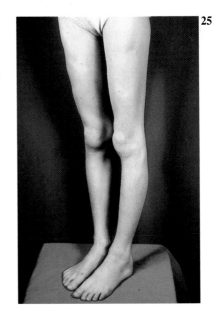

26 (a) What defect does this infant demonstrate?
(b) In what syndrome is this occasionally seen?

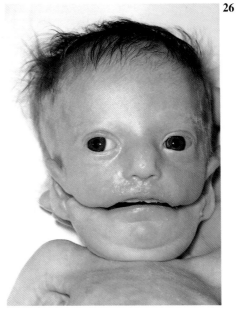

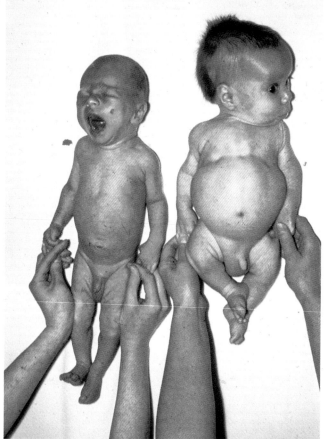

27 The infant on the left of these two newborn infants of the same gestational age is normal.
(a) What condition does the other infant have?
(b) What is the mode of inheritance?
(c) What spinal lesion is often a feature of this condition?

28 A nine-year-old boy developed bilateral parotid swelling and neck stiffness following a two-day history of pain in the angle of the jaw and general malaise. Examination of the CSF showed 400 lymphocytes per mm^3.

(a) What condition is the boy suffering from?

(b) What may be revealed by clinical examination of the throat?

(c) Name two further complications of the primary illness.

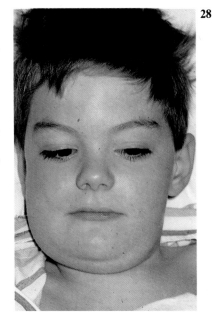

29 This five-year-old girl had been unwell with a swinging pyrexia for one week.

(a) What is demonstrated?

(b) What diagnosis does this physical sign suggest?

(c) Name the two investigations of choice to prove the most likely diagnosis.

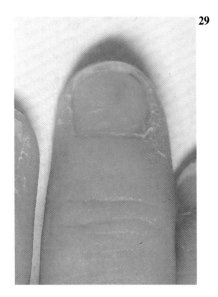

30

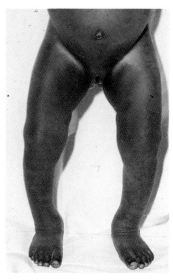

30 A health visitor noticed the features shown in a routine examination of toddlers attending a nursery.

(a) What gave cause for concern?

What is the likely explanation for the finding:

(b) in an asymptomatic child?

(c) in a child reared in a poor social environment?

(d) in a child known to be suffering from chronic renal disease?

31 This baby was noted to have two cutaneous abnormalities at birth.
(a) What are they?
(b) What early investigation should be performed?

31

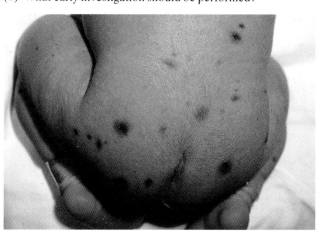

32 A three-year-old boy was referred because of psychomotor delay. Chromosomal examination revealed a deletion of the short arm of chromosome 5.
(a) What is the diagnosis?
(b) Name two characteristic features shown that suggest the diagnosis.
(c) What is the prognosis for height and longevity?

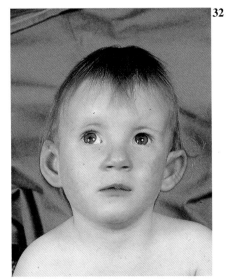

33 Radiograph of a one-month-old infant who had received intensive care in the neonatal period.
(a) What abnormality is shown?
(b) What is the likely cause?

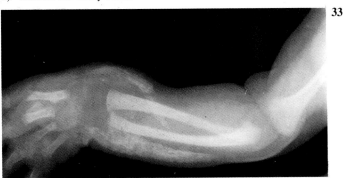

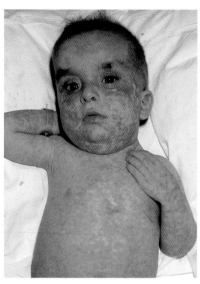

34 A six-month-old infant was admitted unwell, with a fever and rash.

(a) Which exanthem is he suffering from?

(b) State three complications of the illness.

(c) If the child developed the rash in an open hospital ward, how should the other patients be managed?

35 An eight-day-old infant was referred for assessment of ambiguous genitalia. There were no other clinical abnormalities. The chromosomes were 46 XY and the plasma 17-OH progesterone was normal. Careful examination of the inguinal canal revealed bilateral undescended gonads.

(a) What is the diagnosis?

(b) Name three investigations that may be helpful.

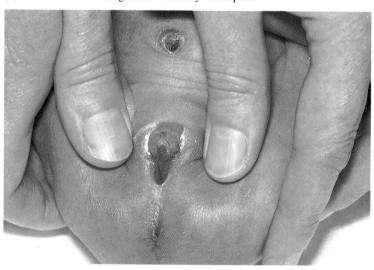

36 This operation was performed on a two-day-old infant who had been noted to have scrotal swelling, during the course of a routine examination.
(a) What is demonstrated?
(b) What additional surgical procedure is essential?

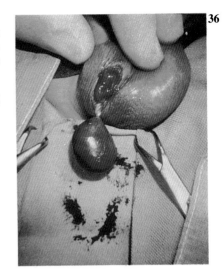

37 A three-year-old boy was referred because of recurrent fever and abnormal dentition. The fevers tended to occur most often during the summer and had been particularly troublesome during the family holiday in Spain. They had not responded to any form of therapy other than tepid sponging. On examination the teeth were noted to be widely spaced and peg-shaped.
(a) What is the diagnosis?
(b) What is the cause of the recurrent fevers?
(c) Name two further complications of this condition.

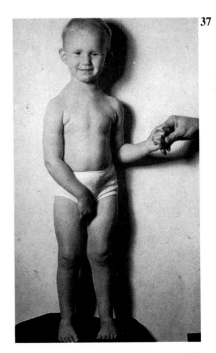

38

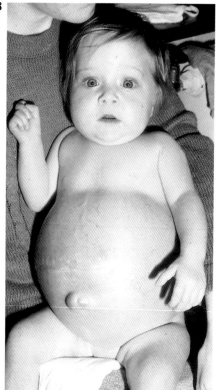

38 (a) Name three clinical abnormalities visible in this nine-month-old child.
(b) What is the likely cause of these abnormalities?
(c) What is the treatment of choice?

39

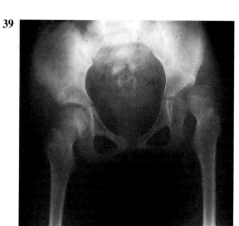

39 This three-year-old child presented with a limp.
(a) What is the diagnosis?
(b) What is the approximate incidence of this condition?

40 This newborn baby shows a striking abnormality.
(a) What is it?
(b) Name three conditions with which this abnormality may be associated.

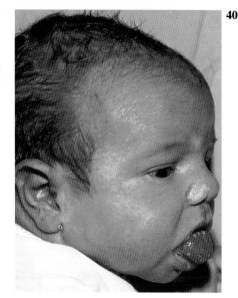

41 This two-year-old presented to the Accident and Emergency Department after a choking attack followed by a six-hour history of acute dyspnoea.
(a) Name three abnormalities seen on the chest radiograph.
(b) What may be the cause?

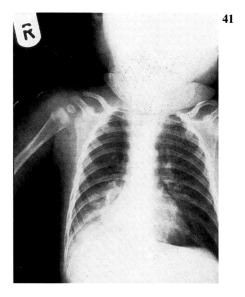

42

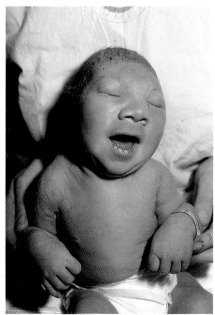

42 (a) What abnormality is seen in this three-week-old infant?
(b) Name one prenatal cause.

43

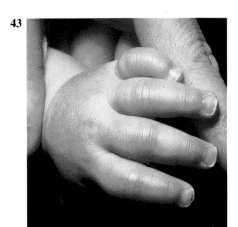

43 This infant had a painful hand.
(a) What abnormality is shown?
(b) Name two causes for the clinical abnormality.

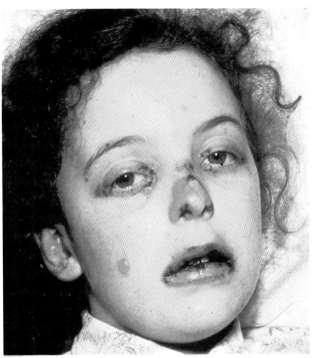

44 This eight-year-old had been treated with cotrimoxazole for her first attack of urinary tract infection. Four days later she presented at the hospital toxic, feverish and with the lesions shown.

(a) What condition is she suffering from?

(b) With what infection may this condition be associated in other patients?

45

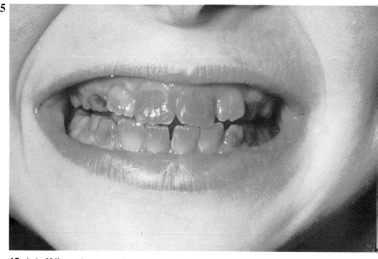

45 (a) What abnormality is shown?
(b) Name two causes of this condition.
(c) After what age is this unlikely to occur?

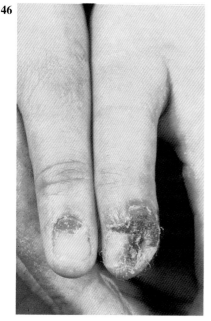

46 A 12-year-old girl was receiving immunosuppressive therapy for a renal disorder. The lesion on her finger had been steadily worsening over the previous two weeks. Initially, her parents felt that it was due to her chewing her nails but later they sought medical advice.
(a) What is the diagnosis?
(b) What is the treatment of choice?

47 This child presented with a long history of vomiting after feeds, which was worsening.
(a) What is demonstrated?
(b) What is the likely aetiology?

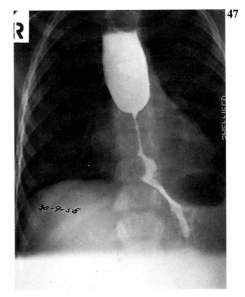

48 An eight-year-old girl presented to her family doctor with a history of fever, sore throat and general malaise, for which she was treated with an antibiotic. Several days later she developed the rash shown.
(a) What is the rash due to?
(b) What was the likely presenting complaint?
(c) Which two laboratory investigations might help in confirming the diagnosis?

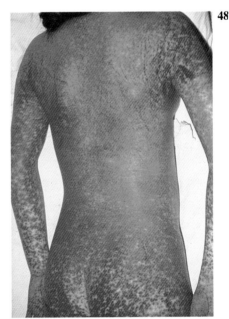

49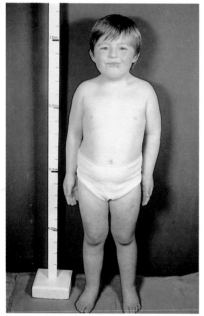

49 This mentally retarded girl under cardiac follow-up for pulmonary stenosis was referred for evaluation of short stature. Chromosome analysis was 46 XX.
(a) What is the diagnosis?
(b) What is the mode of inheritance?

50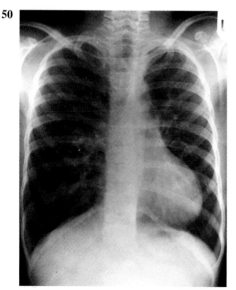

50 This is a radiograph of an eight-year-old boy with a systolic murmur.
(a) List two abnormalities.
(b) What is the likely diagnosis?

51 (a) What abnormality is present in this radiograph of a two-year-old?
(b) What is the most likely cause?

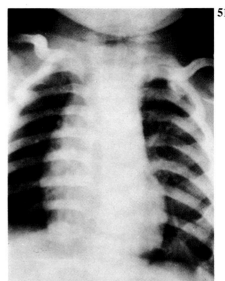

52 A three-year-old child presented to her family doctor with a history of proptosis, gradually worsening over the past three weeks. On examination a mass in the left flank was palpated.
(a) What is the diagnosis?
(b) Name three investigations that should be carried out.

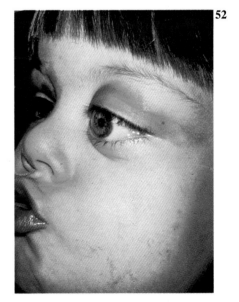

53

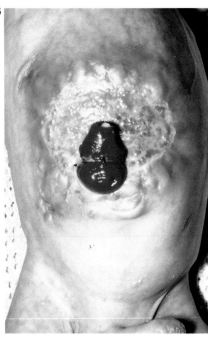

53 (a) What is demonstrated here?

(b) What is the likely cause of the excoriation present?

54

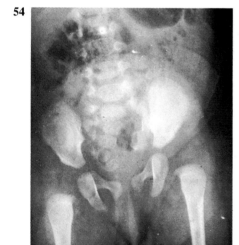

54 A two-day-old infant was referred because of an abdominal mass. On examination he was noted to have a smooth suprapubic mass, dribbling of urine and a patulous anus. A cleft was present over the left side of the sacrum.

(a) What is demonstrated in the radiograph?

(b) What is the abdominal mass?

(c) What is the diagnosis?

55 The facies of this newborn infant are characteristic of a chromosomal anomaly.

(a) What is the condition called and which chromosomes are abnormal?

(b) What abnormality of the feet is often seen?

(c) What is the long term prognosis?

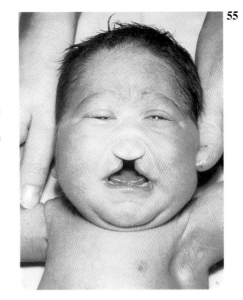

56 (a) What is the diagnosis?

(b) What is the commonest immediate complication?

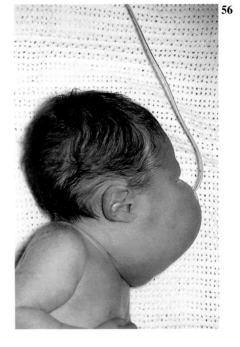

57

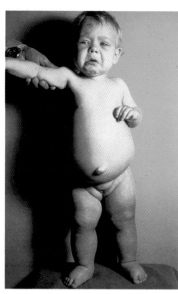

57 A two-year-old child presented with generalised oedema; examination of the urine showed marked proteinuria but no haematuria.

(a) What condition is she likely to suffer from?

(b) What percentage of such children will relapse?

(c) What is the treatment of choice?

58 (a) What abnormality can be seen in this newborn baby?

(b) What is the anatomical defect?

(c) In what syndrome is this often found?

58

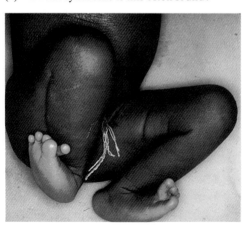

59 A child was admitted to hospital moribund suffering from septicaemia. The skin lesions shown appeared over the next 48 hours during treatment in the intensive care unit.
(a) What is the nature of the lesions?
(b) What is the commonest cause in childhood for this sequence of events?

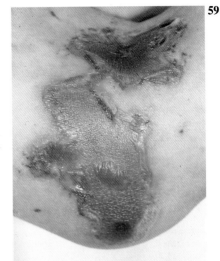

60 (a) What abnormalities are present in this newborn infant?
(b) What is the likely diagnosis?
(c) What is the inheritance?

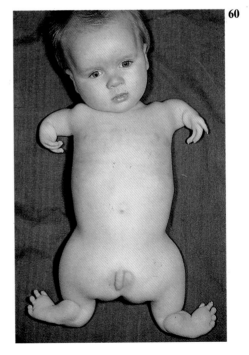

61

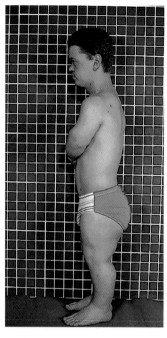

61 This is a picture of a 14-year-old boy.
(a) What is the likely diagnosis?
(b) What cervical spine abnormality may be present in this condition?

62

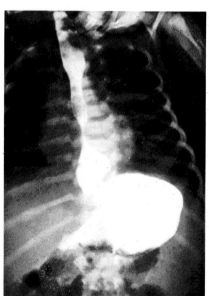

62 A barium meal was performed on an 18-month-old boy who presented with a history of persistent vomiting.
(a) What abnormality is demonstrated on this radiograph?
(b) Name three other common presentations for this condition in childhood.

63 A five-year-old girl presented with recurrent abdominal pain and bloody diarrhoea.
(a) What abnormalities are apparent in the perineal region?
(b) The lesions and the history are characteristic of which condition?
(c) What is the investigation of choice?

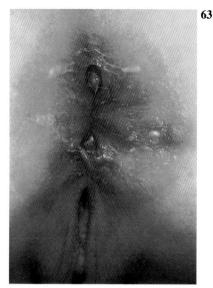

64 Skull radiograph of a child who had a history of focal convulsions.
(a) What abnormality is shown?
(b) What is the mode of inheritance of the underlying condition?

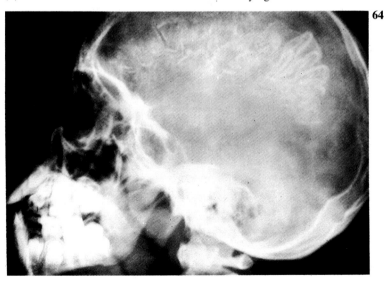

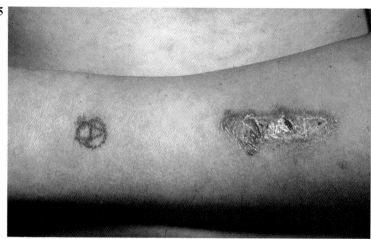

65 This is the forearm of a 14-year-old girl who has a disturbed family background.
(a) What lesions are shown?
(b) What is the likely cause of the inflamed lesion?

66 A seven-year-old boy was referred to Outpatients because of difficulty in micturition.
(a) What lesion is shown?
(b) What is the treatment?

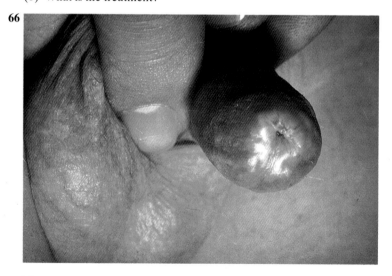

67 This is a computerised axial tomogram of a three-month-old baby.
(a) What abnormality is present?
(b) What facial features may co-exist?

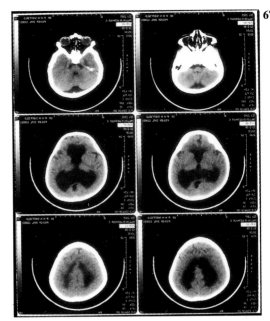

68 This is a radiograph of a four-day-old infant who presented with poor feeding and breathlessness. He was not cyanosed.
(a) Give three abnormalities demonstrated on the film.
(b) What is the probable diagnosis?

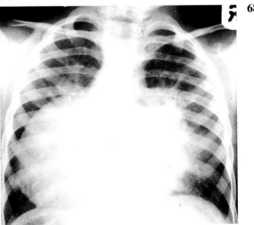

69

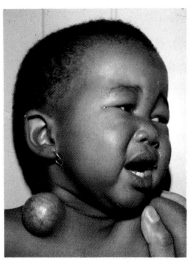

69 A child of African parents presented with a three months' history of progressive malaise, weight loss and nocturnal cough. The swelling was first noticed one month after the onset of symptoms. Examination revealed an unwell child with an enlarged inflamed right tonsil but no other abnormality.

(a) What is the most likely diagnosis?

(b) Name two investigations that may be useful.

70 This is a picture of an infant aged two hours.
(a) What is the diagnosis?
(b) What is the function of the cling film?
(c) How is this condition most commonly diagnosed?

70

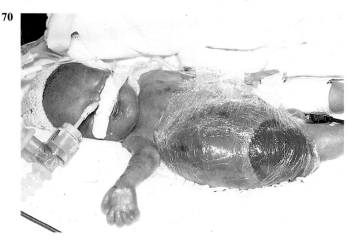

71 A child was noted to have a neck swelling at school entry examination which moved when she stuck out her tongue. Between referral and attendance at Outpatients she developed malaise, a swinging fever and tenderness over the lump.
(a) What is the diagnosis?
(b) What is the treatment of choice?

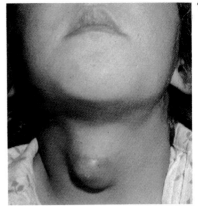

72 This is a picture of a four-year-old girl.
(a) What is demonstrated?
(b) How may this be caused?

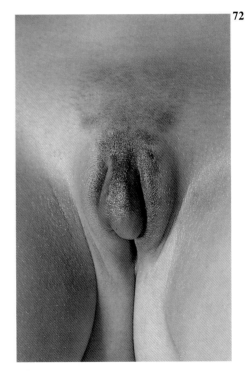

73

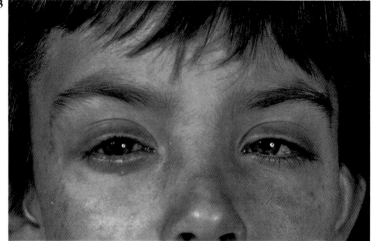

73 A five-year-old girl was under neurological supervision for progressive ataxia. At a clinic visit her mother pointed out the facial rash which had not responded to topical ointment prescribed by her general practitioner.
(a) What is the diagnosis?
(b) What is the mode of inheritance?
(c) Name two serious long term complications.

74

74 This is a radiograph of a newborn infant with respiratory distress.
(a) What is demonstrated?
(b) Give two possible aetiologies.

75 Radiograph of a five-year-old boy with a chronic cough that did not respond to repeated courses of antibiotics. His parents reported that he had fed well from birth but had gained weight slowly. Examination showed him to be below the 3rd centile for height and weight. Auscultation of the chest showed bilateral basal crepitations.
(a) What abnormality is seen in the radiograph?
(b) What is the most likely diagnosis?
(c) If the likely diagnosis is confirmed, what test should be carried out on his two-year-old sister?

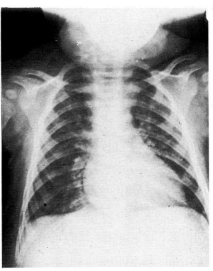

75

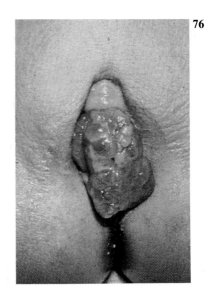

76

76 A little girl presented with acute urinary retention.
(a) What abnormality is shown?
(b) What age range is most commonly affected?
(c) How is this condition treated?

77

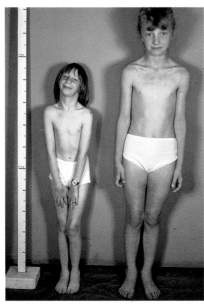

77 A larger than average seven-year-old girl is shown with a patient.
(a) Name three abnormalities visible in the patient.
(b) What is the possible diagnosis?
(c) What is the prognosis for final stature?

78

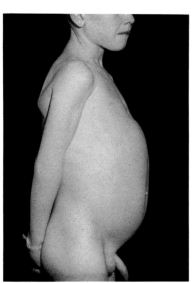

78 A 10-year-old boy presented with a history of gross constipation since early life. Treatment with laxatives had been largely ineffective.
(a) What abnormality is shown?
(b) What is the most likely diagnosis?
(c) What is the treatment of choice?

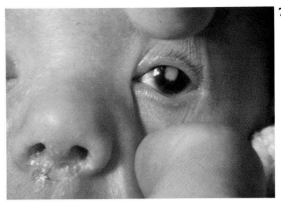

79 (a) What abnormality is apparent in this one-month-old infant?
(b) Name three possible causes in this particular case.

80 Specimen of brain and spinal cord taken from a short child who died suddenly, having been asymptomatic up to the moment of death.
(a) Describe the two abnormalities demonstrated.
(b) What was the child's likely primary pathology?

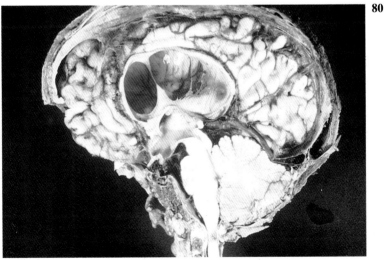

80

81

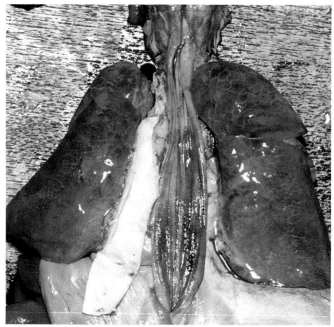

81 (a) What abnormality is shown?
(b) What is the commonest reason for this?

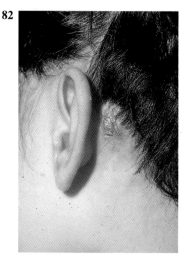

82 An 11-year-old boy presented to Outpatients with this lesion which had been present for eight months and discharging purulent material for six weeks. The lesion appeared after the boy had hurt himself in a swimming pool on holiday in the USA. Despite topical therapy the lesion had increased in size. A swab from the ulcer grew no bacteria after 48 hours but a 1:1000 Mantoux test produced a 7mm diameter reaction.
(a) What is the likely diagnosis?
(b) What is the treatment of choice?

83 This picture shows a barium study of a 12-year-old with weight loss and vomiting.
(a) What is demonstrated?
(b) What is the likely diagnosis?
(c) In which protozoal infection may similar findings be seen?

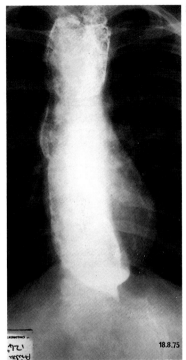

84 (a) What abnormality is shown in this nine-month-old infant?
(b) In what syndrome may this occur?
(c) What is the treatment of choice?

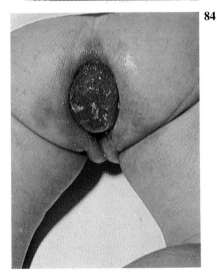

85

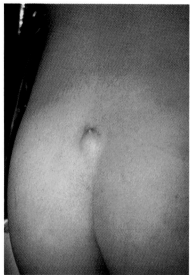

85 (a) What physical condition can be seen in this three-year-old?
(b) Name four common causes.

86

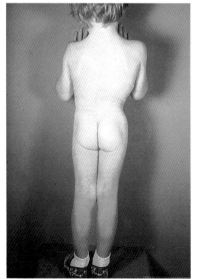

86 An eight-year-old child presented with acute paralysis of both legs associated with loss of bladder and bowel control. The lesion shown had been present since birth, but had been asymptomatic.
(a) What is the lesion?
(b) What emergency investigation should be carried out?

87 A rash was noted on a four-day-old baby.
(a) What is the most likely cause?
(b) What is the differential diagnosis?

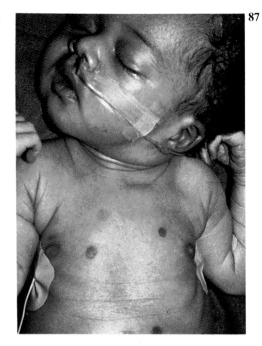

88 A four-year-old boy arrived at the Accident and Emergency Department three hours after having been stung by a wasp.
(a) What is the diagnosis?
(b) What is the treatment of choice?

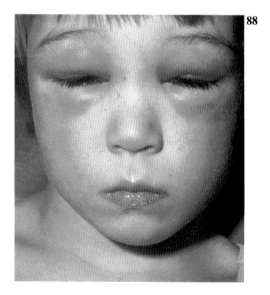

89

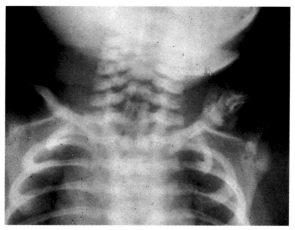

89 This is a picture of a two-week-old infant.
(a) What abnormality is shown?
(b) How may this present?
(c) What treatment is necessary?

90 (a) What condition is this?
(b) What is the cause?
(c) What clinical symptoms and signs may be associated with this abnormality?

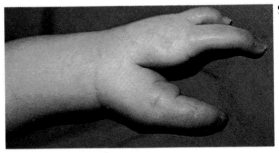

91 (a) What defect is this?
(b) In what syndrome is this abnormality characteristic?
(c) With which other feature is it associated?

92 This nine-month-old baby, thought to be normal at birth, was grossly macrosomic when reviewed.
(a) Give three possible causes.

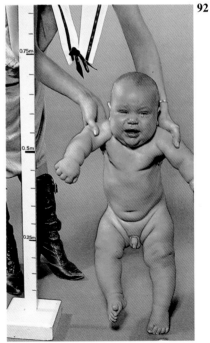

93

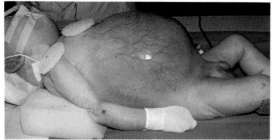

93 (a) Describe the abnormality apparent in this five-day-old infant.
(b) Name four causes.

94

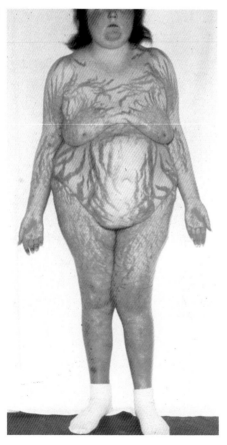

94 A 10-year-old girl presented with distressing obesity, and a careful history failed to reveal any evidence of drug ingestion.
(a) What is the likely diagnosis?
(b) What effect is this likely to have on her adult height?
(c) What is the commonest aetiology in this child?

95 A midwife found it impossible to take a rectal temperature reading after removing a meconium-filled nappy.
(a) What is the likely explanation for this?
(b) What is the treatment of choice?

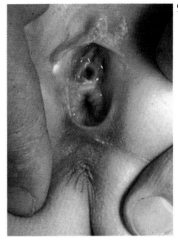

96 (a) What abnormality is seen in this baby's facial structure?
(b) With what tumour is this phenomenon sometimes associated?

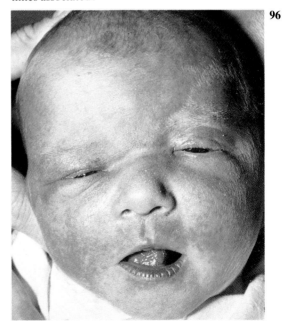

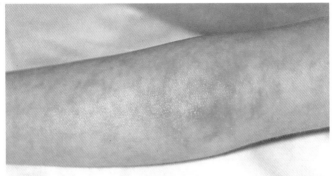

97 This six-year-old girl presented with weakness, an abnormal gait and this rash over her elbow.
(a) What is the diagnosis?
(b) What abnormality may be present on the face?
(c) What is the treatment of choice?

98 These infants are twins photographed within one hour of birth.
(a) What condition is illustrated?
(b) Which of the twins is at greater risk?
(c) What treatment is required?

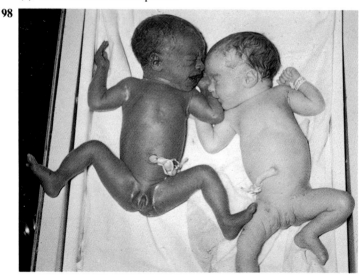

99 An 18-month-old boy was born large-for-dates and macroglossia was apparent at birth. He was operated on in the immediate neonatal period for exomphalos.

(a) What condition is he suffering from?

(b) What abnormality of the ears is characteristic of this syndrome?

(c) In what way may such infants have a life-threatening crisis?

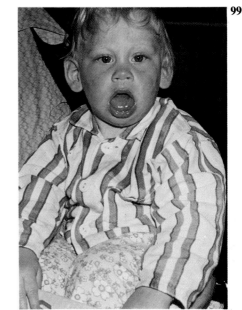

100 A newborn infant was noted to have this lesion present from birth. Name three possible diagnoses.

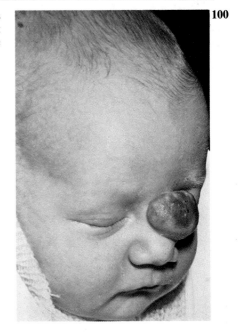

101

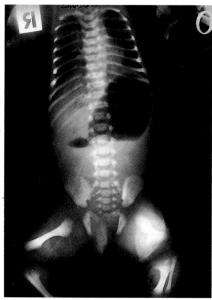

101 This is a radiograph of a vomiting newborn infant.
(a) What is the diagnosis?
(b) In what chromosomal disorder is this more frequently seen?
(c) What accounts for the appearance of the left leg?

102

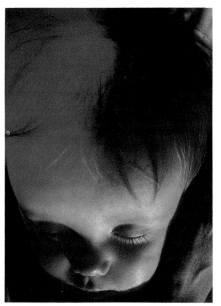

102 These are the results of transillumination of the skull of a three-month-old infant.
(a) What abnormality is shown?
(b) Name two possible causes.

103 This child presented with a limp.
(a) What abnormality is demonstrated?
(b) What is the diagnosis?
(c) What is the appropriate therapy?

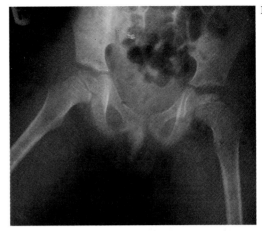

104 A four-week-old infant was the third child of healthy, unrelated parents. Pregnancy and delivery were uncomplicated and the baby was discharged home well at the age of 48 hours. He presented with a lump in the neck.
(a) What is the diagnosis?
(b) What is the treatment of choice?
(c) How commonly does this occur following uncomplicated delivery?

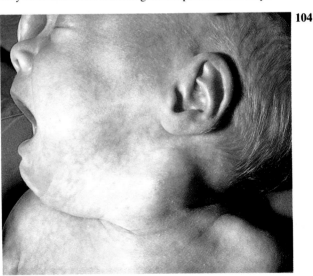

105

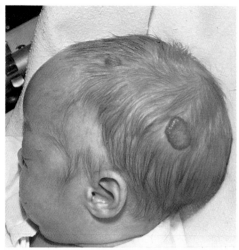

105 (a) What condition is shown?
(b) In what circumstances may surgical removal of the lesion be indicated?

106

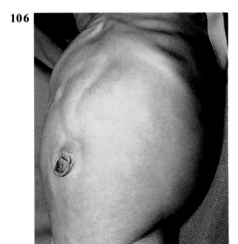

106 A five-week-old infant presented with a three-day history of vomiting. The vomitus was not bile-stained. The infant was constipated.
(a) What abnormality is seen in this illustration which was taken at the time of a test feed?
(b) What is the likely diagnosis?
(c) What abnormality of acid-base balance may be found and how should it be treated?

107 An asymptomatic newborn baby has a chubby leg.
(a) Is it abnormal?
(b) If so, why and with what condition may it be associated?

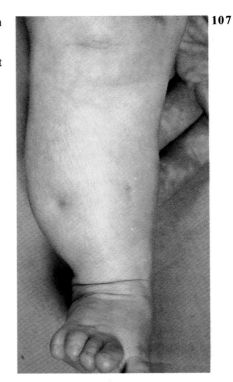

108 (a) What is wrong with this baby's umbilicus?
(b) What is the cause?

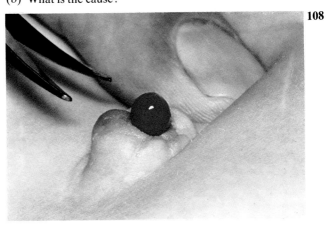

109

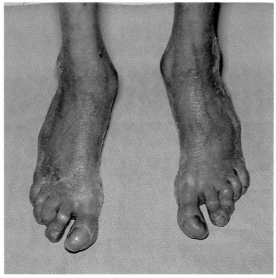

109 This is a picture of the feet of a 13-year-old.
(a) What abnormalities are present?
(b) What is the likely diagnosis?

110 This baby was born at term to a healthy mother. Chromosomal examination was 46 XX. The serum 17 alpha hydroxyprogesterone level was markedly raised.
(a) What is the diagnosis?
(b) What is the mode of inheritance?
(c) What percentage of such children will be predisposed to electrolyte abnormalities?

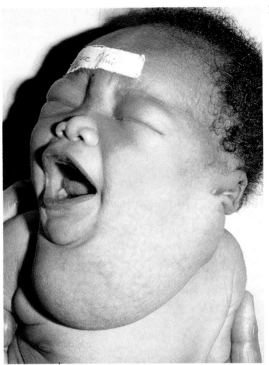

111 (a) What abnormality is demonstrated by this baby?
(b) What side effects may occur shortly after birth?

112 (a) What abnormality is seen in this infant's eyes?
(b) Of what disorder is the abnormality characteristic?

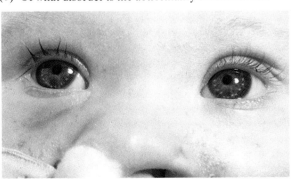

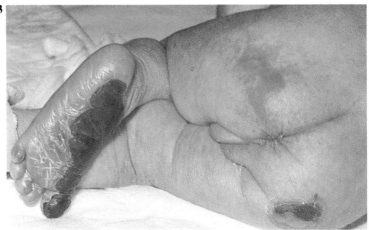

113 This premature infant had received neonatal intensive care and the lesions shown are iatrogenic.
(a) What procedure is likely to have been carried out?
(b) What is the pathogenesis of the lesions?

114 A 12-year-old presented with gradual loss of vision.
(a) What is the diagnosis?
(b) How is this condition usually inherited?

114

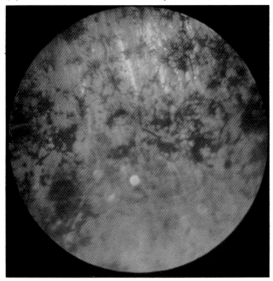

115 (a) What is the diagnosis in this picture?
(b) How may this be suspected clinically?

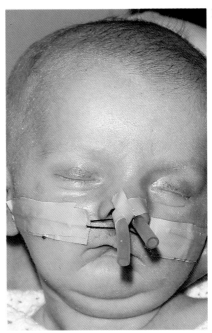

116 A newborn infant attracted attention because of her feet.
(a) What is wrong?
(b) With what systemic abnormality is this sign characteristically associated?

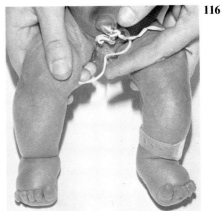

117

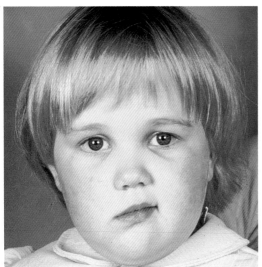

117 A two-year-old girl on antimitotic therapy for acute lymphoblastic leukaemia suddenly developed this lesion.
(a) What is the diagnosis?
(b) Name two possible aetiological factors.

118 (a) What physical signs are demonstrated in this knee?
(b) What is the likely underlying cause?

118

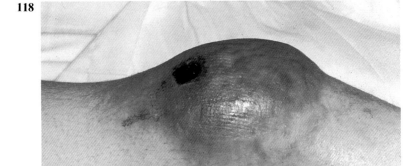

119 A seven-year-old girl was referred from the School Health Service because of short stature. Her progress in school was satisfactory and her parents had no specific worries. Her weight was on the 50th centile, her height was on the 3rd. Both parents were on the 75th centile for height.

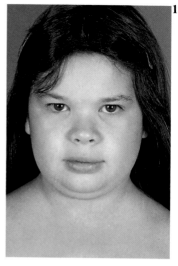

(a) What is the diagnosis?
(b) In children presenting in this way, is school progress normally satisfactory?
(c) State two investigations that will help you to arrive at a diagnosis.

120 A five-month-old boy presented with a dermatitis that had not responded to conventional topical treatment. On examination he had a similar eruption on the scalp and severe otitis externa. The liver was enlarged to 5 cm and splenomegaly was present. A full blood count revealed a haemoglobin of 8g%, white cell count 1,200 with a differential of 60% neutrophils, 30% lymphocytes, 7% monocytes, 2% eosinophils, 1% basophils. The platelet count was 95,000 per cu.m.

(a) What is the likely diagnosis?
(b) How may this be proven most easily?

120

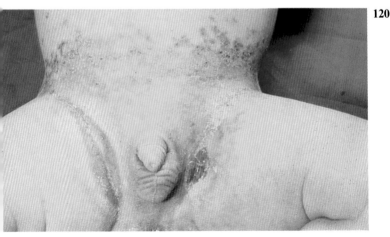

121

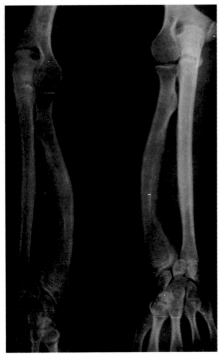

121 (a) What is the diagnosis in this picture?
(b) In what systemic condition is it frequently seen?
(c) What treatment is available?

122

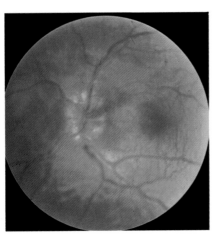

122 (a) Name three abnormalities seen in this fundus.
(b) Name four possible causes for these findings.

123 (a) Identify two abnormalities in this 11-year-old boy.
(b) What is the diagnosis?
(c) How is the condition
inherited?

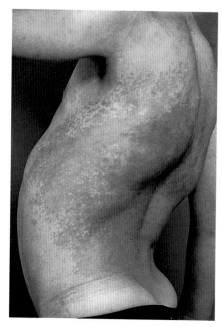

124 A two-year-old child was referred to an orthoptic clinic because of
squint which had developed in the previous two weeks. Examination
revealed paralysis of the right lateral rectus muscle.
(a) How should the child be managed?
(b) What underlying cause may account for this?

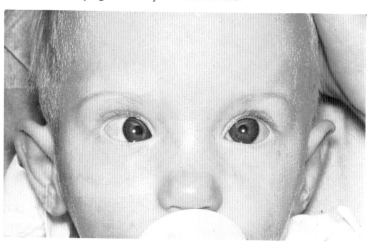

125 Radiographs demonstrate views obtained on a barium swallow examination performed on a child with recurrent vomiting and pneumonia.
(a) What is shown?
(b) What is the likely anomaly?

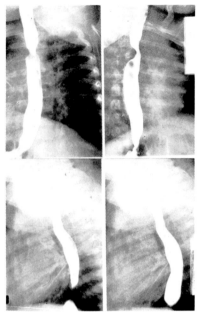

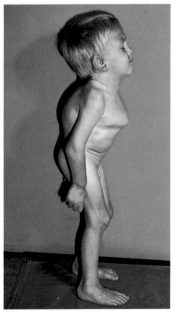

126 A six-year-old boy of normal intelligence has an inborn error of metabolism resulting in skeletal deformity.
(a) What is the diagnosis?
(b) What is the inheritance?
(c) What is the laboratory investigation of choice?

127 This is a picture of an eight-month-old infant. In addition brachysyndactyly was present.
(a) What is the diagnosis?
(b) Which sutures are predominantly affected?
(c) What is the mode of inheritance?

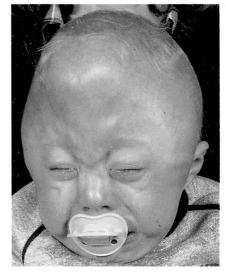

128 (a) What abnormality is shown?
(b) Name three syndromes in which this may occur.

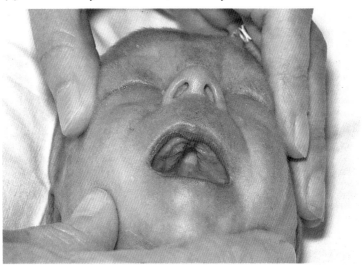

129 Concern was expressed about this 22-hour-old baby boy.
(a) What abnormality is shown?
(b) What is this due to?
(c) What is the prognosis for long term continence of stool?

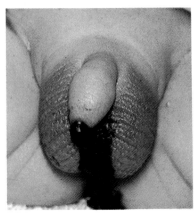

130 This is the postmortem appearance of an 11-year-old child who had been slightly off-colour for one week. The family doctor had noted purulent tonsillitis and had prescribed penicillin. One afternoon after returning from swimming she felt faint and complained of shoulder pain. She became rapidly pale and shocked and was dead on arrival at the hospital.
(a) What was the immediate cause of death?
(b) What may have been the underlying illness?

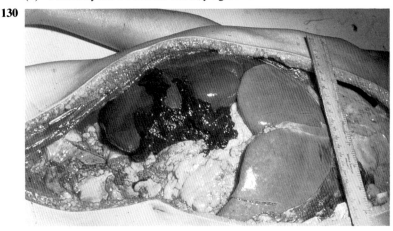

131 An 18-month-old child was born at 28 weeks' gestation and required prolonged neonatal intensive care.
(a) What abnormality is shown?
(b) What may have been the cause?

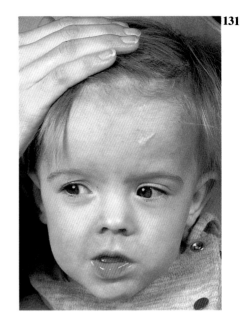

132 This skin lesion appeared spontaneously in this two-day-old baby. A similar lesion appeared on the hand. The child appeared well and active otherwise.
(a) What is the diagnosis?
(b) How is this normally inherited?
(c) What is the prognosis?

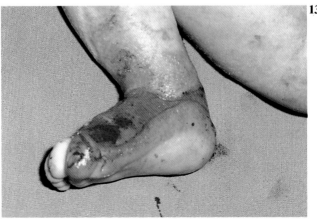

133

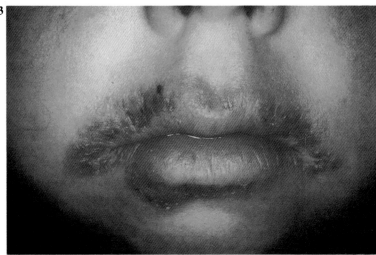

133 A four-year-old boy was noted to develop discoloration of his lips two months prior to acute admission to hospital with severe abdominal pain and melena. Similar lesions were noted on his mother's lips but she was asymptomatic.
(a) What is the diagnosis?
(b) What treatment is usually required?
(c) What is the main complication of this condition?

134

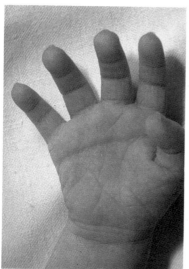

134 This is the hand of a one-year-old infant with developmental delay.
(a) Name two abnormalities.
(b) What is the likely diagnosis?
(c) What endocrine abnormality is more frequent in this syndrome?

135 An eight-year-old girl was referred because of short stature.
(a) What three abnormalities are seen?
(b) What is the diagnosis?
(c) How many children with this condition enter spontaneous puberty?

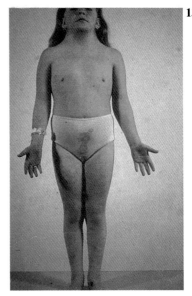

136 (a) What is apparent in this small intestinal wall?
(b) Name three possible causes.

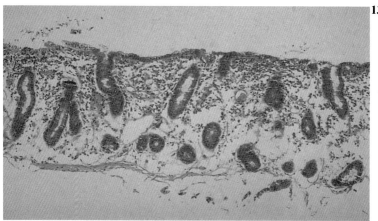

137

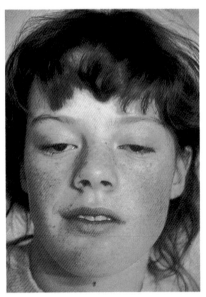

137 A 13-year-old girl presented to Outpatients with a six-month history of muscle weakness which worsened as the day progressed. Her family doctor had thought she was suffering from hysteria. Referral was prompted by the development of diplopia.
(a) What physical sign is shown?
(b) What is the most likely diagnosis?
(c) How may this be confirmed?

138 (a) What abnormality does this child demonstrate?
(b) In what syndrome is this found?

138

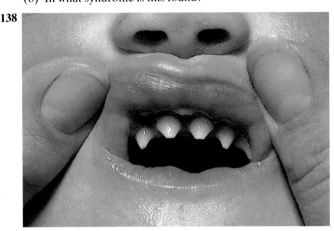

139 A six-month-old infant was admitted to hospital for plastic surgery.
(a) What condition is shown?
(b) How is this inherited?

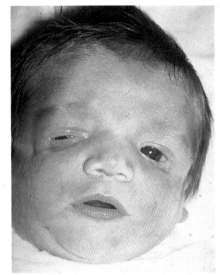

139

140 This is the CAT scan of a three-year-old admitted with blindness, cerebral palsy and macrocephaly.
(a) Describe the abnormalities seen in the scan.
(b) Suggest a possible pathophysiology and diagnosis.

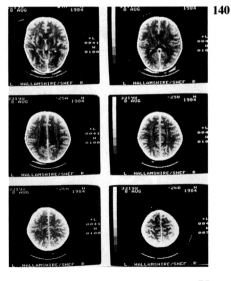

140

141

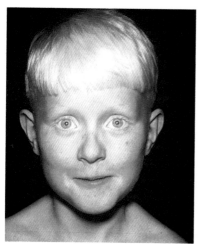

141 (a) What is wrong with this boy?
(b) What is the mode of inheritance?

142 (a) What condition does this child have?
(b) What clinical feature does this have in common with osteogenesis imperfecta?
(c) Name two other common findings.

142

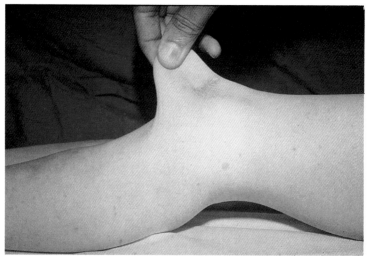

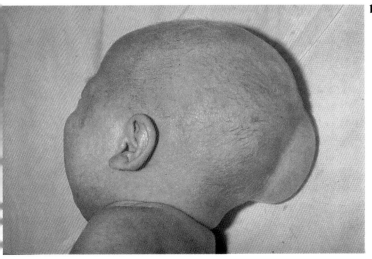

143 An eight-week-old infant presented with a lump on the head. Name three important differential diagnoses.

144 This is the picture of a two-day-old infant.
(a) What abnormalities are seen in the lower limbs?
(b) What is the likely cause?

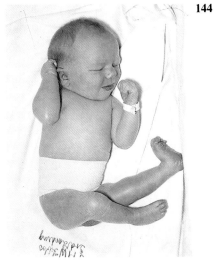

145

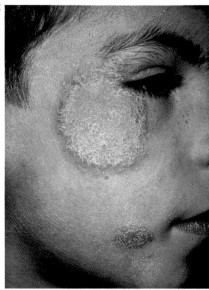

145 (a) What lesion shown on this girl's face?
(b) What is the treatment of choice?

146

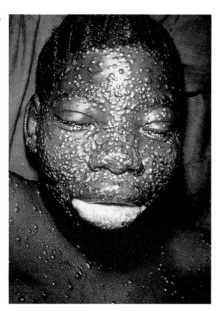

146 A 10-year-old boy presented to a mission hospital with severe headache, back ache and the above rash.
(a) What is the diagnosis?
(b) What abnormality is characteristic in the white cell count?
(c) What is the incubation period?

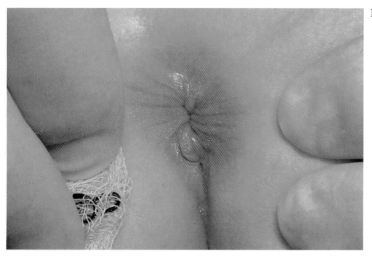

147 This three-year-old presented to outpatients with screaming on defaecation and bright red blood in the stools.
(a) What is the diagnosis?
(b) What is the treatment of choice?

148 (a) What abnormality is shown in this 11-year-old girl?
(b) What is the likely diagnosis?
(c) What ocular complication may be found?

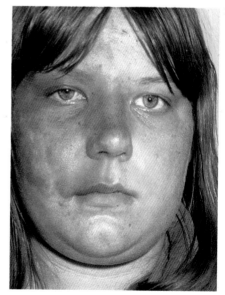

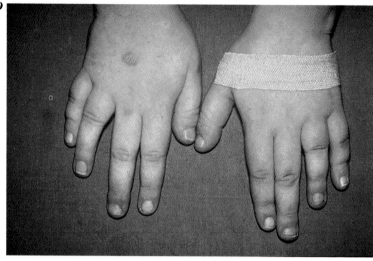

149 The hands of a five-year-old boy referred for assessment of growth failure and mental retardation.
(a) What abnormality is shown?
(b) What is the diagnosis?
(c) Name three other possible clinical findings.

150 A two-month-old infant was referred because of poor feeding. On examination he was noted to hold his head retracted and to have persistent flexion of the arms and legs. When questioned his mother said this had always been the case.
(a) What is the most likely diagnosis?
(b) Name three causes with origin in the neonatal period.

151 A three-year-old girl became ill one week previously when the only clinical abnormality was an abrasion on the cheek. This subsequently ulcerated with gradual development as shown, despite ampicillin treatment.
(a) What abnormality is seen?
(b) What is the likely causative organism?
(c) What is the treatment of choice?

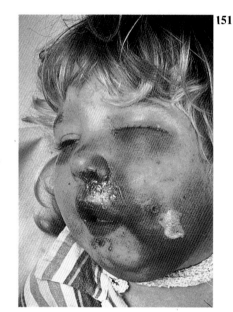

152 This is a lateral radiograph of the lower legs of a nine-year-old boy.
(a) What abnormality is present?
(b) In what systemic disease is this often found?
(c) What is the major complication of the defect?

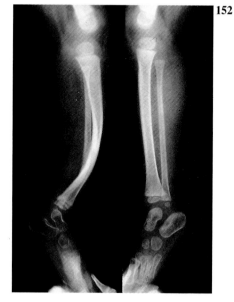

153

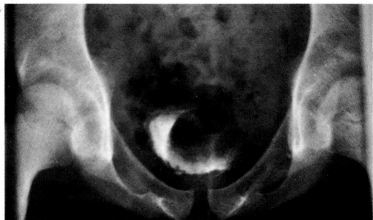

153 This radiograph was obtained during excretory urography of a six-year-old girl being investigated for recurrent urinary infection.
(a) What abnormality is shown?
(b) How is it caused?

154 This is the neck of a nine-year-old girl who presented in Dermatology outpatients. Her brother had been treated for a similar eruption two months earlier.
(a) What is the diagnosis?
(b) What is the aetiology?
(c) What is the prognosis without treatment?

154

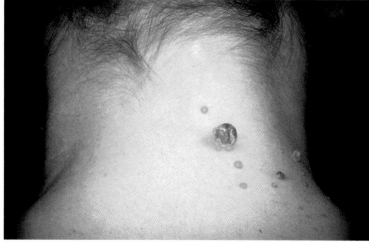

155 This child presented with failure to thrive and neurological retardation.
(a) What abnormality is present?
(b) What is the diagnosis?
(c) How is the condition inherited?

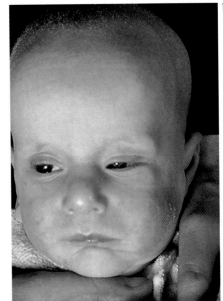

156 This is a slide of a short, mentally retarded five-year-old girl.
(a) List two abnormal features.
(b) What is the likely diagnosis?

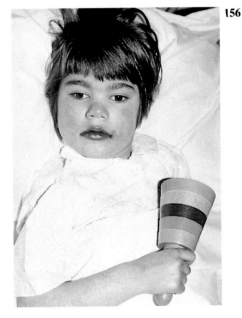

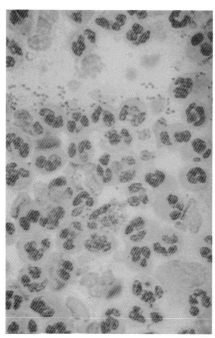

157 The microscopic appearance of CSF from a three-year-old child admitted with fever and neck stiffness.
(a) Name two abnormalities shown.
(b) What is the diagnosis?
(c) What is the treatment of choice?

158 The patient is a 16-year-old boy.
(a) What abnormal clinical signs are present?
(b) How may they be explained?

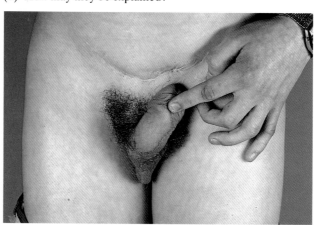

159 A 12-year-old girl was referred because of progressively deteriorating school performance.
(a) What abnormalities can be seen?
(b) What is the diagnosis?
(c) What is the treatment of choice?

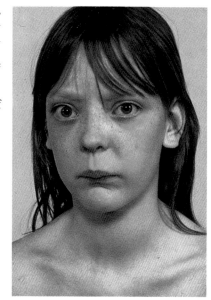

160 Radiograph of a four-year-old child with abdominal distension of three months' duration.
(a) What examination is being performed?
(b) What abnormality is demonstrated?
(c) What is the most likely cause?

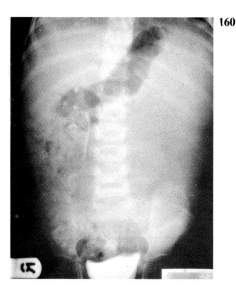

161

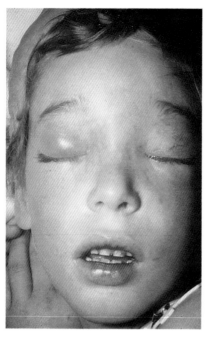

161 A five-year-old boy had a purulent nasal discharge for one week which had been treated with decongestants. The day before admission to hospital he developed a fever and drowsiness. He progressed rapidly to the appearance shown at the time of admission to hospital.
(a) What is the diagnosis?
(b) What is the treatment of choice?
(c) What may be revealed by examination of the CSF?

162

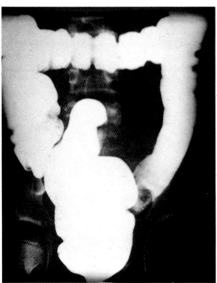

162 (a) Name two abnormalities seen in this radiograph of a barium enema examination.
(b) What is the diagnosis?
(c) Name the treatment of choice.

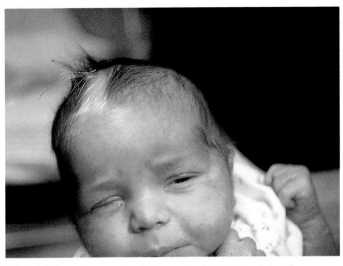

163 (a) What abnormality is demonstrated in this picture?
(b) What is the diagnosis?
(c) Name two additional abnormalities likely to be present.

164 A four-year-old boy was referred because of developmental delay. Clinical examination revealed small nails, an ejection systolic murmur in the aortic area and a height and weight each below the 3rd centile. A radiograph of the wrist for the determination of bone age revealed increased bone density as a coincidental finding.
(a) What abnormalities can be seen?
(b) What is the diagnosis?
(c) What is the likely cause of his cardiac murmur?

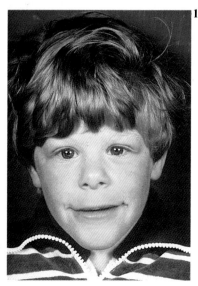

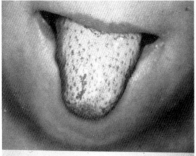

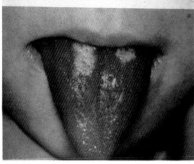

165 (a) What abnormalities are shown in these tongues?
(b) In what condition may they be seen?
(c) What is the treatment of choice for this condition?

166 A three-year-old girl was hospitalised because of a severe persistent cough.
(a) What abnormality is shown?
(b) What is the likely cause of her illness?

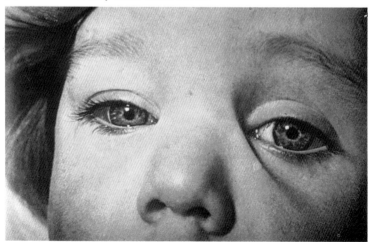

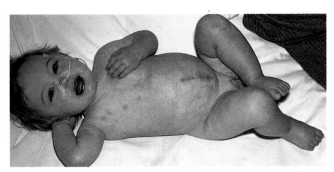

167 A two-year-old was transferred from another hospital for further investigation. She had been febrile, unwell and had generalised abdominal tenderness. Laparotomy revealed no abnormality. Two days later she developed this rash and generalised lymphadenopathy. On arrival at the referral centre, conjunctivitis, stomatitis and erythema of the hands and feet were also noted. Her fever continued to spike over the next week when peeling of the hands and feet occurred.

(a) What is the diagnosis?
(b) Name three further complications.
(c) What is the likely cause of her abdominal pain?

168 This is a picture of two brothers. The parents became concerned when the younger boy became taller than his sibling.

(a) What is the likely diagnosis?
(b) What is the approximate frequency of this condition?

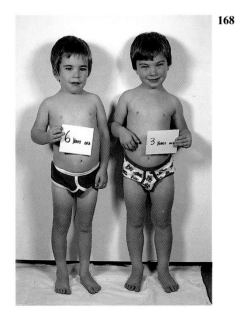

169

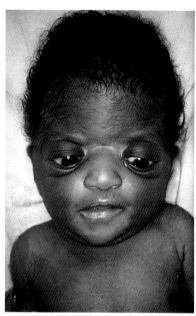

169 A two-year-old boy was referred to the Outpatient clinic because of his unusual appearance and failure to thrive. On examination he was noted to have broad thumbs and cryptorchidism.

(a) What abnormalities can be seen?

(b) What is the diagnosis?

(c) What is the prognosis for growth and for mental development?

170

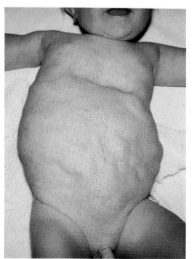

170 (a) What syndrome is demonstrated?

(b) Name two clinical problems associated with this.

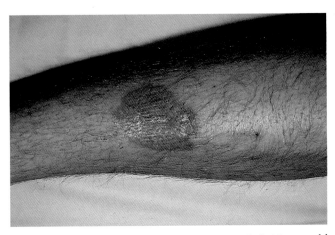

171 This lesion presented in a well controlled 15-year-old diabetic boy.
(a) What is the diagnosis?
(b) What treatment is available?

172 This is the picture of the legs of an eight-month-old infant.
(a) What abnormality is demonstrated?
(b) Name three clinical features with which this phenomenon may be associated.

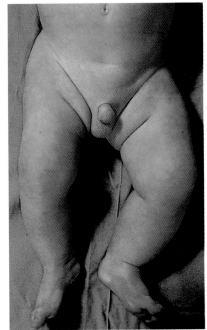

173 This radiograph was performed on an eight-year-old child.
(a) What is demonstrated?
(b) Describe an important clinical feature of the condition.

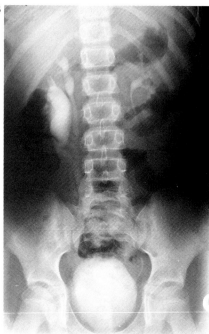

174 This is a radiograph of a 12-year-old.
(a) What is the diagnosis?
(b) With what may this be associated?

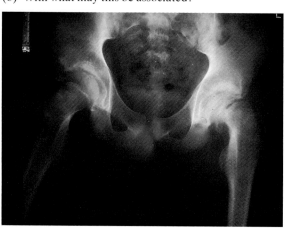

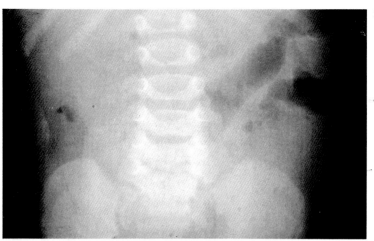

175 This is the plain abdominal radiograph of a three-year-old child who had been well until the previous day. Following an episode of diarrhoea she had intermittent attacks of abdominal pain and pallor. The general practitioner thought an abdominal mass was present but this was not confirmed by the casualty officer.
(a) What lesion is shown?
(b) What is the treatment of choice?
(c) What other modes of treatment are available?

176 This boy presented with acute difficulty in micturition.
(a) What condition is shown?
(b) What is the treatment of choice?

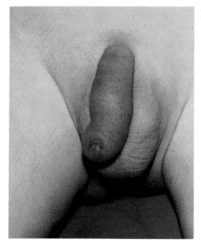

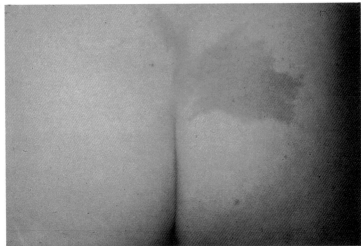

177 A two-year-old girl seen in Orthopaedic outpatients because of bowing of the legs was referred to the medical Paediatric clinic because of early breast development. Additionally, the abnormal skin pigmentation shown was noted. A similar lesion was present on her neck.
(a) What is the diagnosis?
(b) How do these lesions differ from those seen in neurofibromatosis?

178 The mother of this two-day-old infant had been regularly taking a proprietary iodine containing preparation, unknown to her attending physicians.
(a) What is the diagnosis?
(b) Give two common complications.

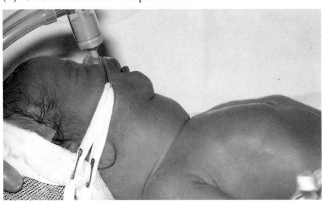

179 (a) What abnormality is shown?
(b) What is the aetiology?
(c) What treatment is available?

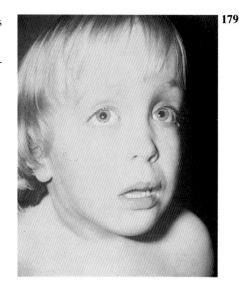

180 (a) What condition is apparent?
(b) Name three pulmonary and three other causes.

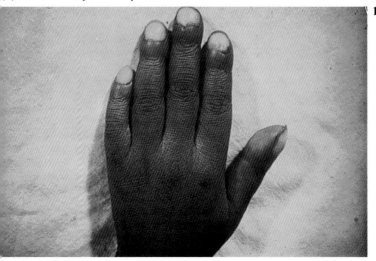

181

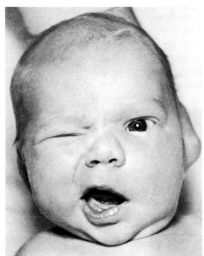

181 (a) What abnormality is shown?
(b) What is the prognosis?

182

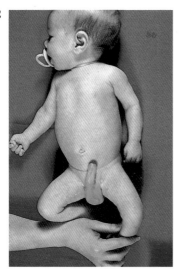

182 (a) What abnormality is present in this five-day-old infant?
(b) What underlying condition must be excluded?

183 (a) What rash is shown?
(b) Name two conditions in which it may occur.

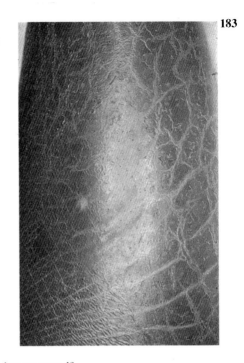

184 (a) What abnormality is demonstrated?
(b) Name three syndromes in which it may be found.

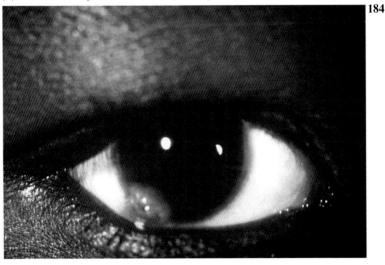

185 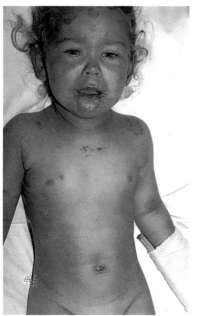 A three-year-old girl presented to her general practitioner with a pustule on the face. This was treated with topical antibiotics. Despite treatment the pustule increased in size before finally bursting. Three days later she developed a fever and erythema of the cheek which spread to the forehead and trunk. The rash then began to exfoliate and this coincided with increasing lethargy, anorexia and fever.
(a) What is the diagnosis?
(b) What is the aetiology of the rash?
(c) What treatment is indicated?

186 (a) What is this lesion?
(b) Name two ocular complications that may be seen.

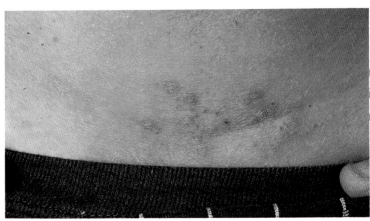

187 An 18-month-old infant presented with a swelling in the sacrococcygeal area of two months' duration. He had also lost weight and been anorexic with a cough. The swelling had increased in size gradually and the child had recently developed urinary retention. Laboratory investigations showed a raised alphafetoprotein and alpha 1 anti-trypsin in the blood.

(a) What is the diagnosis?
(b) What is the likely cause of the cough?

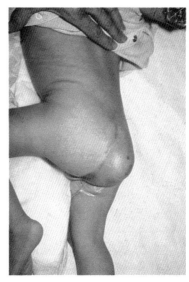

188 (a) What abnormality is shown?
(b) Name two syndromes in which this may occur.

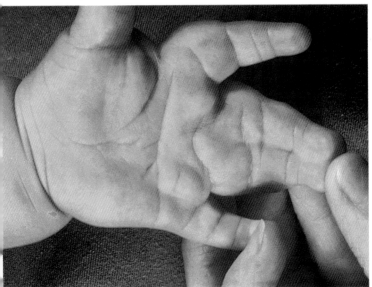

189

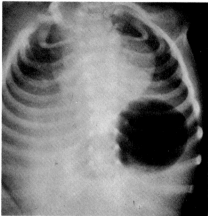

189 Radiograph of a one day-old infant who had vomited all feeds.
(a) Name three abnormalities shown.
(b) What is the likely cause of the abnormalities?

190 A 12-year-old boy was referred to a neurologist because of deteriorating school performance and increasing clumsiness. He also had the rash shown, moderate ataxia, hearing loss and retinal findings similar to those seen in retinitis pigmentosa. He deteriorated and six months later was unable to walk.
(a) Name the rash.
(b) What is the likely cause of the neurological deterioration?
(c) What treatment is available?

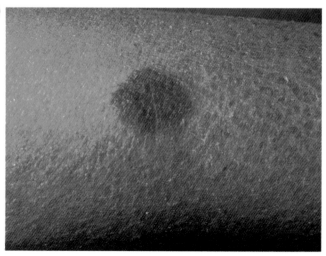

191 What is demonstrated in this picture?

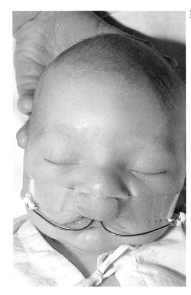

192 This is a picture of a 12-year-old boy with emotional problems.
a) What is demonstrated?
b) What is the probable diagnosis?
c) What side effect may be seen in affected females?

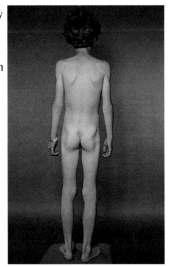

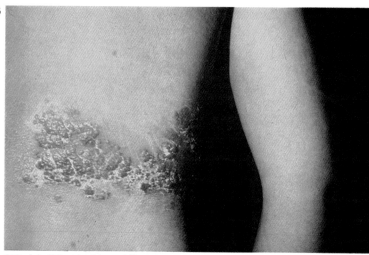

193 (a) What is this rash?
(b) What is the aetiology?
(c) How long does it take to resolve?

194 Radiograph of a two-year-old child of Asian parents who presented with a history of weight loss and cough.
(a) What abnormalities are shown?
(b) What is the likely diagnosis?
(c) What two investigations will be of benefit?

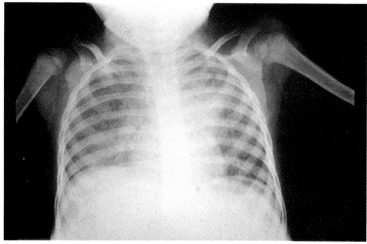

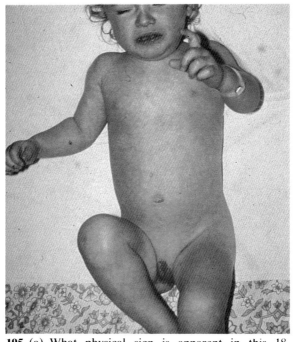

195 (a) What physical sign is apparent in this 18-month-old girl?
(b) Name three investigations of value in establishing the diagnosis.

196 (a) What physical sign is seen in this eight-year-old girl?
(b) Name two important causes.

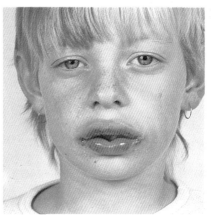

197

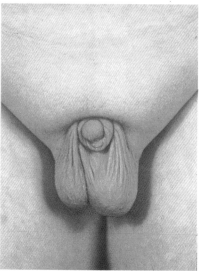

197 A nine-year-old boy presented to Outpatients because of school avoidance, particularly on days when he was due to have a P.E. lesson.
(a) What is the reason for his school phobia?
(b) State three possible causes.

198 A special investigation was performed on a two-year-old who presented with increasing weakness of the left leg.
(a) What investigation has been performed?
(b) What is demonstrated?
(c) What is the diagnosis?

198

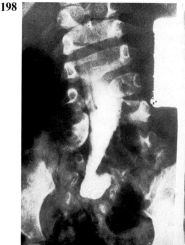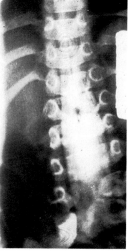

199 This is an illustration of a two-year-old girl.
(a) What abnormality is shown?
(b) Give two possible aetiologies.

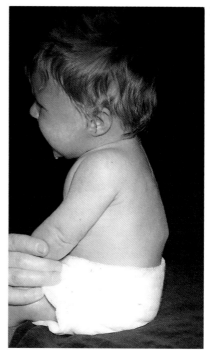

199

200 What is the aetiology of this lesion?

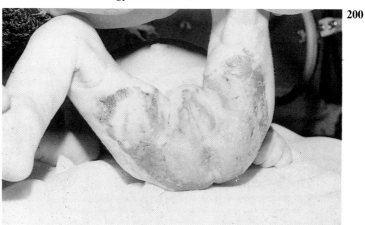

200

201

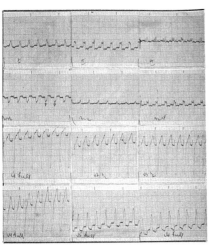

201 Cardiogram of a four-year-old presenting with shock and peripheral shutdown.
(a) What is demonstrated?
(b) What is the likely underlying cardiac lesion?

202 These lesions were noted on the scalp of a newborn baby.
(a) What are they?
(b) In which syndrome are they commonly found?
(c) What is the investigation of choice?

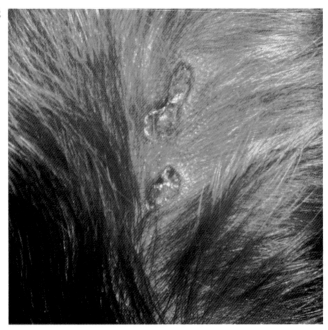

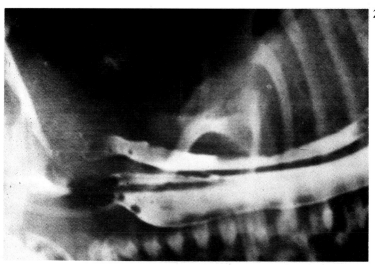

203 This radiograph shows a special investigation being performed on a three-month-old infant with recurrent wheeze.
(a) What is the investigation?
(b) What is demonstrated?
(c) What is the diagnosis?

204 (a) What is the diagnosis?
(b) What is the function of the radio-opaque marker on the skin?

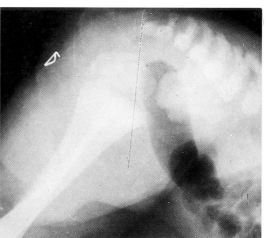

205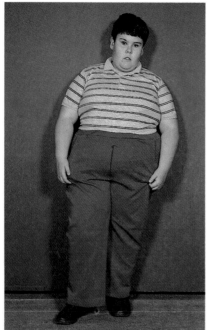
This 14-year-old mentally retarded boy presented with short stature and an insatiable appetite.

(a) What is the most probable diagnosis?

(b) What special investigation may help to confirm this?

206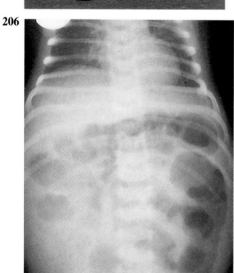
This infant presented at the age of three days with abdominal distension and no history of having passed meconium.

(a) What is demonstrated in this erect radiograph?

(b) What is the differential diagnosis?

207 A six-month-old infant was referred from a surgical clinic where he had been seen for repair of inguinal herniae. His length and weight had been noted incidentally to be below the 3rd centile, and his facial appearance had given cause for concern.

(a) What abnormalities are shown?

(b) What is the diagnosis?

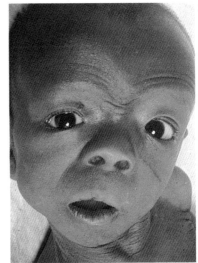

208 CAT scan of a five-month-old child who presented with convulsions, hypotonia and delayed motor milestones. What two abnormalities are present?

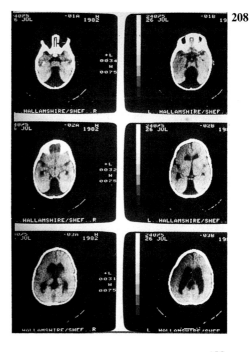

ANSWERS

1 (a) Bilateral ventricular dilation with periventricular brightness, suggesting leukomalacia.
(b) The prognosis for long term development is uncertain, and advice should be guarded.

2 (a) Eczema herpeticum, otherwise known as Kaposi's varicelliform eruption.
(b) Topical and systemic acyclovir. Systemic antibiotics may be indicated if bacterial superinfection is suspected.

3 (a) Erythema multiforme.
(b) The scalp.
(c) None — the rash is self-limiting.

4 Hypotonia at this age may be due to: Down's syndrome, birth asphyxia, hypothyroidism, prematurity, dystrophia myotonica, or maternal benzodiazepine administration.

5 (a) A pseudocyst of the pancreas.
(b) Following abdominal trauma.
(c) An abdominal mass.

6 (a) Severe dental decay.
(b) Improved dental hygiene and avoidance of sugar containing syrups in children requiring long term drug therapy.

7 The film is typical of sickle cell disease. In it are seen sickle cells, target cells, anisocytosis and hypochromia.

8 (a) Situs inversus.
(b) Kartagener's syndrome.
(c) Sinusitis and bronchiectasis.

9 (a) Chicken pox.
(b) Giant cells in scrapings from the lesion; virus culture; rise in antibody titre.

10 (a) Sirenomyelia, also known as 'mermaid' baby.
(b) Before four weeks' gestation.

11 (a) Russell-Silver dwarfism.
(b) Light-for-dates; short stature; hemihypotrophy.

12 (a) Acute osteomyelitis.
(b) Drainage of the infected area, bed rest, immobilisation of the ankle and up to six weeks' parenteral antimicrobial therapy.
(c) Staph Aureus, H Influenzae, M Tuberculosis, Salmonella spp.

13 (a) Von Willebrand's disease.
(b) Decreased Factor VIII concentration; decreased platelet adhesion; impaired platelet aggregation in the presence of ristocetin.

14 (a) Atrophic glossitis.
(b) Iron deficiency, pernicious anaemia, pellagra, tropical sprue.

15 (a) Seborrhoeic dermatitis.
(b) Staphylococcus aureus or Candida albicans.
(c) The scalp.

16 (a) Herpangina.
(b) Coxsackie virus infection.
(c) Treatment is supportive, with particular attention to topical and systemic analgesia.

17 (a) Short trunk compared to overall height.
(b) Structural disease of the spine, spinal radiotherapy.

18 (a) Right atrial enlargement, pulmonary artery dilation, increased pulmonary vascularity.
(b) Ostium secundum atrial septal defect.
(c) Right axis deviation, right ventricular hypertrophy, right bundle branch block.

19 (a) A parotid abscess.
(b) Mumps.
(c) Staphylococcus aureus.

20 (a) Thoracic dystrophy.
(b) Autosomal recessive.

21 (a) The sex of the child—Hurler's syndrome is inherited as an autosomal recessive; Hunter's as an X-linked recessive.
(b) Nodules over the scapula are found in Hunter's but not in Hurler's syndrome.
(c) A cloudy cornea is found in Hurler's but not in Hunter's syndrome.

22 (a) Herpes stomatitis.
(b) Gentian violet has been applied topically.
(c) Application of topical acyclovir.

23 (a) Bronchography.
(b) Sequestration of the left lower lobe.

24 (a) Crohn's disease.
(b) Stomatitis.
(c) Barium meal and follow-through.

25 (a) Diabetic lipoatrophy.
(b) Lipoatrophy (and hypertrophy) can be lessened by rotation of injection site and by use of monocomponent insulin preparations.

26 (a) Midline facial cleft.
(b) Goldenhar's syndrome.

27 (a) Achondroplasia.
(b) Inheritance is an autosomal dominant.
(c) Kyphosis.

28 (a) Mumps.
(b) Displacement of the tonsils towards the midline.
(c) Further complications include pancreatitis and orchitis.

29 (a) Splinter haemorrhages.
(b) Subacute bacterial endocarditis.
(c) Blood culture; cardiac ultrasound looking for vegetations.

30 (a) Bow legs.
(b) No cause discoverable.
(c) Vitamin D deficient rickets.
(d) Renal rickets.

31 (a) Lentigines (big freckles) and a Mongolian blue spot.
(b) Hearing test to exclude the multiple lentigines syndrome.

32 (a) Cri-du-chat syndrome.
(b) Hypertelorism and prominent ears.
(c) Adult height is reduced but longevity is unaffected.

33 (a) Subcutaneous calcification.
(b) This was a complication arising from subcutaneous leakage of calcium being given intravenously.

34 (a) Measles.
(b) Complications include encephalitis, pneumonitis and subacute sclerosing panencephalitis.
(c) Other hospitalised patients in contact should be given protective immunoglobulin injections, if they are immunodeficient or under the age of nine months. Otherwise they should be vaccinated against measles immediately if this has not been done.

35 (a) Intersex.
(b) Rectal examination for palpation of the cervix, laparoscopy and/or pelvic ultrasound to identify the internal genitalia, and gonadal biopsy to determine whether or not one or both gonads is an ovotestis.

36 (a) Torsion of the testis.
(b) The other testis should be operated on also to prevent the occurrence of torsion.

37 (a) Anhydrotic ectodermal dysplasia.
(b) Absence of sweat glands.
(c) Recurrent pulmonary infections, atrophic rhinitis, dysphonia.

38 (a) Jaundice, a caput medusa and abdominal swelling with an umbilical hernia.
(b) Biliary atresia.
(c) Treatment is surgical and involves anastomosis of the duodenum to the porta hepatis.

39 (a) Congenital dislocation of the left hip.
(b) 1:1400.

40 (a) A protruding tongue.

(b) Down's syndrome, hypothyroidism and the Beckwith-Wiedemann syndrome.

41 (a) Mediastinal shift, a hyperexpanded left lung and consolidation in the right middle and lower lobes.
(b) These findings together with the history are compatible with the aspiration of a foreign body.

42 (a) Microcephaly.
(b) Congenital infection, eg by rubella or cytomegalovirus. Associated with spina bifida. Sporadic.

43 (a) Dactylitis.
(b) This is commonly caused by juvenile rheumatoid arthritis or by sickle cell disease.

44 (a) Stevens-Johnson syndrome.
(b) Mycoplasma pneumoniae.

45 (a) Staining of the teeth.
(b) The two commonest causes are hyperbilirubinaemia in the neonatal period and tetracycline treatment.
(c) Eight years, although hyperbilirubinaemia may affect the first permanent molars.

46 (a) Monilial paronychia.
(b) Oral griseofulvin with the option of a topical antifungal agent.

47 (a) Oesophageal stricture.
(b) Gastro-oesophageal reflux, which may be associated with hiatus hernia.

48 (a) An ampicillin rash.
(b) Infectious mononucleosis (glandular fever).
(c) Monospot test; abnormal lymphocytes in the peripheral blood smear.

49 (a) Noonan's syndrome.
(b) Usually sporadic.

50 (a) Left ventricular enlargement; rib notching.
(b) Coarctation of the aorta.

51 (a) Healing fracture of the posterior aspect of the ninth right rib.
(b) This finding immediately suggests non-accidental injury.

52 (a) The child has a retro-orbital metastasis of tumour, most probably a neuroblastoma.
(b) Ultrasound examination of the abdomen, whole body CAT scan and biopsy of the mass.

53 (a) Ileostomy.
(b) Leakage of gastrointestinal contents.

54 (a) An intraspinal mass displacing the sacrum.
(b) An enlarged bladder.
(c) An intraspinal tumour, probably a sacral lipoma or dermoid.

55 (a) Patau's syndrome; this is due to trisomy 13.
(b) The feet are often rockerbottom in shape.
(c) The long term prognosis is poor; the patients usually die before the age of one year.

56 (a) Cystic hygroma.
(b) Airway obstruction.

57 (a) Nephrotic syndrome.
(b) Approximately 70%.
(c) Glucocorticoids.

58 (a) Rockerbottom feet.
(b) A vertical talus.
(c) Edward's syndrome.

59 (a) Skin necrosis and sloughing due to disseminated intravascular coagulation.
(b) Meningococcal septicaemia.

60 (a) Phocomelia: marked shortening of the limbs and digital reduction abnormalities.
(b) Thanatophoric dwarfism.
(c) Probable autosomal recessive.

61 (a) Achondroplasia.
(b) Atlanto-axial instability.

62 (a) Hiatus hernia.
(b) Failure to thrive; recurrent chest infections; anaemia.

63 (a) Inflammation of the perineal region accompanied by a fistula.
(b) Crohn's disease.
(c) A barium meal and follow-through examination.

64 (a) 'Railroad' calcification of the cerebral blood vessels due to Sturge-Weber syndrome.
(b) Inheritance is sporadic.

65 (a) A self-inflicted tattoo and dermatitis artefacta.
(b) The girl scraping the skin on her arm.

66 (a) He is suffering from phimosis.
(b) Circumcision.

67 (a) Holoprosencephaly.
(b) Central facial developmental defects such as cleft lip, micropthalmia, nasal abnormalities.

68 (a) Bilateral ventricular enlargement, pulmonary plethora, narrow pedicle.
(b) Truncus arteriosus.

69 (a) Tuberculous cervical lymphadenopathy.
(b) Mantoux test and excision biopsy of the swelling.

70 (a) Exomphalos or gastroschisis.
(b) To prevent heat and insensible fluid loss from the exposed gut.
(c) By antenatal ultrasound screening in mothers performed because a raised serum alphafetoprotein has been found on routine screening.

71 (a) Infected thyroglossal cyst.
(b) Antibiotic therapy initially, followed by excision of the cyst.

72 (a) Perineal bruising with oedema of the labia majora.
(b) Direct trauma; sexual interference.

73 (a) Ataxia telangiectasia.
(b) Inheritance is autosomal recessive.
(c) Increased frequency of infection due to immunological deficiency; increased incidence of brain tumours.

74 (a) Pneumoperitoneum; the viscus outlined is the liver.
(b) From perforation of the gastrointestinal tract or downward tracking of air from a pneumothorax or pneumomediastinum.

75 (a) Numerous areas of patchy consolidation with bronchial wall thickening.
(b) Cystic fibrosis.
(c) A sweat test.

76 (a) Sarcoma botryoides due to a rhabdomyosarcoma of the vagina.
(b) Infants of less than one year.
(c) Surgery and radiotherapy.

77 (a) Microcephaly, a large nose and shortness.
(b) Seckel's bird-headed dwarfism.
(c) Adult height is markedly reduced in those who survive.

78 (a) Marked abdominal distension.
(b) Hirschsprung's disease.
(c) Treatment will probably involve a colostomy followed by resection of the affected segment and a pull-through operation.

79 (a) A cataract.
(b) A cataract found at the age of one month could be due to Down's syndrome, galactosaemia or congenital rubella.

80 (a) Hydrocephalus and compression of the cervical cord.
(b) Achondroplasia.

81 (a) The pathological specimen shows corrosive oesophagitis.
(b) This is most commonly the result of accidental ingestion of a corrosive substance such as caustic soda (lye).

82 (a) Atypical mycobacterium infection.
(b) Excision possibly with antituberculous chemotherapy cover.

83 (a) Marked dilatation of the barium-filled oesophagus.
(b) Achalasia of the cardia.
(c) Chaga's disease (American trypanosomiasis).

84 (a) A rectal prolapse.
(b) This should alert the clinician to consider cystic fibrosis.
(c) Treatment is by gentle manual replacement if this does not occur spontaneously.

85 (a) Scoliosis.
(b) It may be congenital, due to spina bifida, neurofibromatosis, or other spinal destructive lesions such as tuberculosis.

86 (a) Spinal dermoid cyst which, in this case, had communicated through a defect in the vertebral arch to the spinal theca.
(b) An emergency myelogram.

87 (a) The lesions are burns from application of a transcutaneous pO_2 monitor.
(b) Includes congenital chicken pox.

88 (a) Angioneurotic oedema.
(b) Adrenalin and/or systemic antihistamines.

89 (a) A fracture of the left clavicle.
(b) An asymptomatic lump with crepitus on palpation.
(c) Usually none.

90 (a) Sprengel's deformity.
(b) Failure of descent of the scapula from the neck resulting in elevation of the shoulder on the affected side.
(c) There may be limitation of abduction of the arm and associated rib and vertebral anomalies.

91 (a) Lobster-claw hand.
(b) It is seen in Cornelia de Lange syndrome.
(c) Cleft lip and palate.

92 (a) Gross overfeeding, Sotos syndrome, growth hormone secreting adenoma.

93 (a) Gross abdominal distension associated with widespread erythema of the anterior abdominal wall.
(b) Necrotising enterocolitis, volvulus, primary peritonitis, or spontaneous perforation of the bowel.

94 (a) Cushing's syndrome.
(b) If untreated, this will result in stunting of final adult height.
(c) It is most likely to be due to a pituitary tumour.

95 (a) The child has an imperforate anus. She has passed meconium through a rectovaginal fistula. In the illustration, the upper opening is the urethra and the lower a common orifice for the vagina and rectum.
(b) A defunctioning colostomy followed by reconstruction of a functioning anus.

96 (a) There is hemihypotrophy, the left side of the face being larger than the right.

(b) Wilms' tumour.

97 (a) Dermatomyositis.
(b) A heliotrope rash around the eyes.
(c) Systemic corticosteroids.

98 (a) The twins are classical examples of the twin-to-twin transfusion syndrome due to an arteriovenous fistula in a common placenta.
(b) The polycythaemic infant.
(c) A modified partial exchange transfusion in which blood is removed and replaced by plasma.

99 (a) Beckwith–Wiedemann syndrome.
(b) There may be a horizontal crease in the ear lobe.
(c) They may suffer hypoglycaemic crises.

100 The lesion could be a nasal encephalocele, a nasal dermoid, or a cavernous haemangioma.

101 (a) Duodenal atresia.
(b) Down's syndrome.
(c) The orientation of the radiograph.

102 (a) A subdural effusion.
(b) This could have occurred as a result of trauma during or after birth or as a result of meningitis.

103 (a) Flattening and distortion of the left femoral head.
(b) Perthe's disease.
(c) Maintaining the femur in abduction using braces or splints while continuing to permit weight bearing.

104 (a) Sternomastoid tumour.
(b) Leave it alone.
(c) They mostly occur following uncomplicated delivery.

105 (a) A cavernous haemangioma of the scalp.
(b) Surgical removal is rarely indicated. If the haemangioma is causing trouble due to bleeding or platelet consumption, surgical treatment by embolisation or thrombosis is preferable.

106 (a) Waves of peristalsis in the epigastrium.
(b) Pyloric stenosis.
(c) The baby is likely to have a metabolic alkalosis and should be treated with intravenous saline and potassium supplements.

107 (a) The abnormality is a dimple over the tibia and fibula.
(b) It is characteristic of hypophosphatasia, a rare condition due to deficiency of alkaline phosphatase which results in failure of calcification of all bones.

108 (a) An umbilical polyp.
(b) This arises when the vitelline duct fails to obliterate and atrophy.

109 (a) Severe contractures of the joints with lateral deviation of the toes and ulceration over pressure areas.
(b) Rheumatoid arthritis.

110 (a) Congenital adrenal hyperplasia, in this case due to 21-hydroxylase deficiency.
(b) Inheritance is autosomal recessive.
(c) Approximately 30% of such patients will have salt-losing crises.

111 (a) A cystic hygroma of the neck, not a goitre.
(b) The lesion may cause pressure symptoms on the trachea.

112 (a) Brushfield spots.
(b) Down's syndrome.

113 (a) Umbilical arterial catheterisation.
(b) The skin necrosis of the right buttock and left foot may be embolic or may follow spasm and thrombosis of the internal obturator artery and femoral artery.

114 (a) Retinitis pigmentosa.
(b) As an autosomal recessive, autosomal dominant or X-linked recessive. The most common inheritance is autosomal recessive.

115 (a) Choanal atresia.
(b) The child will be cyanosed when not crying.

116 (a) Lymphoedema of the feet and legs.
(b) This is a classical sign of Turner's syndrome.

117 (a) Seventh nerve palsy.
(b) Meningeal infiltration by leukaemic cells, a bleed into the central nervous system due to thrombocytopenia, neuropathy associated with vincristine therapy.

118 (a) Haemarthrosis of the knee.
(b) This is most likely to be due to Factor VIII deficiency or haemophilia.

119 (a) Juvenile myxoedema.
(b) Surprisingly, such patients are commonly said to have satisfactory school progress because of their placidity.
(c) Investigations of value include a serum thyroxine, TSH and a radiological determination of bone age.

120 (a) Histiocytosis X.
(b) By histological examination of a skin biopsy.

121 (a) Madelung's deformity.
(b) Leri-Weill's disease.
(c) Corrective osteotomy.

122 (a) Blurring of the optic disc, fundal haemorrhage and tortuosity of the vessels.
(b) Hypertension, intracranial neoplasm, intracranial haemorrhage, meningitis, or other causes of raised intracranial pressure.

123 (a) A large neurofibroma and lordo-scoliosis.
(b) Neurofibromatosis.
(c) Inheritance is autosomal dominant.

124 (a) Acute onset paralysis of any external ocular muscle requires vigorous investigation for the cause.
(b) Examples of lesions resulting in external rectus paralysis are: intracranial tumour, neurodegenerative disorders.

125 (a) Indenting of the oesophagus due to extramural pressure.
(b) A vascular ring.

126 (a) Morquio's syndrome.
(b) Autosomal recessive.
(c) A key investigation is examination of the urine for keratan and chondroitin sulphate.

127 (a) Carpenter's syndrome.
(b) Coronal, but the lambdoid and sagittal sutures may also fuse early.
(c) Autosomal recessive.

128 (a) A cleft of the soft and hard palate not associated with hare lip.
(b) Pierre Robin, Patau's, Opitz, orocraniodigital syndromes.

129 (a) Meconium is being passed per urethrum.
(b) A rectourethral fistula complicating anorectal agenesis.
(c) Poor.

130 (a) Splenic rupture.
(b) This may have occurred as a complication of infectious mononucleosis.

131 (a) Scar on the forehead.
(b) This was due to a drip which had tissued.

132 (a) Epidermolysis bullosa simplex.
(b) Autosomal dominant.
(c) The tendency to blister improves with time and the prognosis is good.

133 (a) Peutz-Jeghers' syndrome.
(b) Supportive.
(c) Malignant change of the bowel polyps.

134 (a) The hand is spade-shaped and shows a single palmar crease and brachydactyly.
(b) Down's syndrome.
(c) Hypothyroidism is more common than in the general population.

135 (a) Webbing of the neck, hypertelorism, increased carrying angle of the arms and widely spaced nipples.
(b) Turner's syndrome.
(c) Approximately 10%.

136 (a) Villous atrophy.
(b) Coeliac disease, tropical sprue, cow's milk protein intolerance, giardiasis, iron deficiency.

137 (a) Ptosis.
(b) Myasthenia gravis.
(c) By reversal of the abnormal clinical signs by intravenous administration of edrophonium chloride.

138 (a) Small, peg-like teeth.
(b) Anhidrotic ectodermal dysplasia.

139 (a) Treacher-Collins syndrome.
(b) Inheritance is autosomal dominant.

140 (a) Cerebral atrophy, derangement and vacuolisation of the white matter.
(b) This is due to spongy degeneration of the white matter, in this case the result of Canavan's disease.

141 (a) He is an albino.
(b) Autosomal recessive.

142 (a) Ehlers-Danlos syndrome.
(b) Blue sclerae are found in both.
(c) Easy bruising and subcutaneous calcification.

143 The lump could be due to a haematoma, abscess or an encephalocoele. An encephalocoele is usually mid-line; the lump appears to be slightly lateral to the mid-line, making this diagnosis less likely.

144 (a) Abnormal posture with hyperextension of the left knee and dorsiflexion of the left ankle. These suggest a lower motor neuron lesion.
(b) Spina bifida.

145 (a) Tinea corporis.
(b) Topical antifungal agents with possible oral griseofulvin.

146 (a) Smallpox.
(b) Neutropenia.
(c) Twelve days.

147 (a) Anal fissure.
(b) Gentle dilatation with possible use of stool softeners.

148 (a) A haemangioma over the maxillary branch of trigeminal nerve.
(b) Sturge-Weber syndrome.
(c) The development of glaucoma.

149 (a) Shortening of the fourth and fifth metacarpals.
(b) This is a characteristic finding in pseudohypoparathyroidism.
(c) Subcutaneous calcification, bowing of the legs, cataracts, thickening of the skull.

150 (a) Cerebral palsy.
(b) Perinatal asphyxia, hypoglycaemia or meningitis.

151 (a) Facial cellulitis.
(b) Staphylococcal infection.

(c) Parenteral flucloxacillin and fusidic acid.

152 (a) Tibial bowing.
(b) Neurofibromatosis.
(c) Fracture with pseudarthrosis formation.

153 (a) A ureterocele.
(b) Ureteric obstruction with consequent ballooning of the distal ureter as it enters the bladder.

154 (a) Molluscum contagiosum.
(b) Infection with a DNA virus of the pox group.
(c) The condition is eventually self-limiting.

155 (a) Abnormal sparse hair.
(b) Menkes' syndrome.
(c) X-linked recessive.

156 (a) Bushy eyebrows that almost meet in the midline; downturning of the upper lip.
(b) Cornelia de Lange syndrome.

157 (a) Numerous pus cells with intracellular and extracellular Gram negative diplococci.
(b) Meningococcal meningitis.
(c) Intravenous penicillin.

158 (a) The boy has secondary sexual characteristics despite an apparently empty scrotum. He also has an abdominal surgical scar.
(b) The commonest explanation would be androgen therapy following castration. In fact, this patient had a functional intra-abdominal testis.

159 (a) A goitre and proptosis.
(b) Thyrotoxicosis.
(c) Carbimazole.

160 (a) Intravenous pyelogram.
(b) The left kidney is non-functioning; there is displacement of the stomach to the right.
(c) Wilms' tumour.

161 (a) Cavernous sinus thrombosis.
(b) Urgent surgical treatment.
(c) Raised pressure, an increase in both the red and white cell count and an elevated protein concentration.

162 (a) Loss of the normal haustrations, and generalised narrowing of the ascending and transverse colon.
(b) Ulcerative colitis.
(c) Initial therapy would include corticosteroids and salazopyrine.

163 (a) The child has a depigmented forelock.
(b) Waardenburg's syndrome.
(c) Deafness, hypopigmentation of the skin and iris.

164 (a) Anteverted nostrils and an elfin facies.
(b) Idiopathic hypercalcaemia (Williams' syndrome).
(c) Supravalvular aortic stenosis.

165 (a) White and red strawberry tongue.
(b) Scarlet fever.
(c) Penicillin.

166 (a) Subconjunctival haemorrhage.
(b) Bordetella pertussis.

167 (a) Kawasaki disease (Mucocutaneous lymph node syndrome).
(b) Encephalitis, arthritis, proteinuria, and arterial aneurysms, particularly affecting the coronary artery.
(c) Mesenteric adenitis.

168 (a) Growth hormone deficiency.
(b) 1:8000, when diagnosed as a primary isolated condition.

169 (a) A prominent forehead, marked epicanthic folds and downward slanting eyes.
(b) Rubinstein-Taybi syndrome.
(c) Somatic growth is poor and most affected patients are mentally handicapped.

170 (a) Prune belly syndrome.
(b) Urinary tract abnormalities and constipation.

171 (a) Necrobiosis lipoidica diabeticorum.
(b) Some improvement may occur after local corticosteroid injection.

172 (a) Hemihypertrophy.
(b) Wilms' tumour, aniridia, hypertrophy of ipsilateral members of paired body organs.

173 (a) Right renal duplex system.
(b) The patient is consistently enuretic by day, but not by night.

174 (a) Slipped femoral epiphysis.
(b) Obesity, particularly in pubertal boys. Growth hormone deficiency.

175 (a) Intussusception.
(b) Hydrostatic reduction.
(c) Surgical excision may be required.

176 (a) Balanoposthitis due to inflammation of the glans and foreskin of the penis extending into the shaft.
(b) Antibiotics followed in some cases by the separation of adhesions.

177 (a) McCune-Albright syndrome (Polyostotic fibrous dysplasia).
(b) The café-au-lait spot in McCune-Albright syndrome has characteristic ragged edges, compared to the smooth edged lesions seen in neurofibromatosis.

178 (a) Congenital goitre.
(b) Respiratory embarrassment as shown here, transient hypothyroidism, difficulty in delivery due to failure of the head to flex.

179 (a) Scaphocephaly.
(b) Premature fusion of the sagittal suture.
(c) Surgical intervention may be indicated if early diagnosis is made.

180 (a) Clubbing.
(b) Cystic fibrosis, lung abscess or bronchiectasis. It may complicate cardiac conditions such as truncus arteriosus or Fallot's tetralogy; it is seen also in cirrhosis of the liver.

181 (a) Complete left facial palsy.
(b) This is usually due to pressure on the facial nerve during forceps delivery. The prognosis for spontaneous recovery is good.

182 (a) Gross enlargement of the penis.
(b) Adrenogenital syndrome.

183 (a) 'Crazy paving' dermatitis.
(b) Kwashiorkor or pellagra.

184 (a) Coloboma of the iris.
(b) Patau's, Goldenhar's and Wolf's syndromes.

185 (a) Ritter's disease.
(b) Staphylococcal exotoxin.
(c) Parenteral cloxacillin and fusidic acid.

186 (a) The rash is a plexiform neurofibroma.
(b) Optic nerve glioma and buphthalmos.

187 (a) A yolk-sac tumour, otherwise known as an endodermal sinus tumour.
(b) Either pulmonary metastases or primary mediastinal involvement.

188 (a) Syndactyly of the third and fourth fingers.
(b) Apert's, Carpenter's or orofaciodigital syndromes.

189 (a) Gastric distension, splaying of the ribs, abdominal distension and no air in the abdomen distal to the stomach.
(b) Complete pyloric obstruction.

190 (a) Ichthyosis.
(b) Refsum's syndrome.
(c) Avoidance of all green plant foods and other phytanic acid containing foods.

191 An infant with a palatal plate in situ, used in the management of cleft lip and palate.

192 (a) Severe loss of subcutaneous fat.
(b) Anorexia nervosa.
(c) Amenorrhoea.

193 (a) Shingles.
(b) Herpes zoster infection.
(c) Spontaneous resolution occurs after 7 to 14 days.

194 (a) Bilateral hilar enlargement, and generalised mottling of both pulmonary fields.
(b) Miliary tuberculosis.
(c) Mantoux test and gastric washings for acid fast bacilli.

195 (a) Pubic hair.
(b) Twenty-four-hour urinary steroid excretion, abdominal ultrasound, abdominal CAT scan and laparoscopy.

196 (a) Inflammation of the lips (cheilitis).
(b) This is seen in febrile illness, contact dermatitis or excess salivation.

197 (a) Embarrassment because of micropenis.
(b) The commonest explanation for this apparent finding is obesity. True micropenis is found in gonadotrophin deficiency and the Prader-Willi syndrome.

198 (a) A myelogram.
(b) Splitting of the lumbar spinal cord by a septum.
(c) A diastematomyelia.

199 (a) An angulated kyphosis, sometimes called a gibbus.
(b) Spina bifida, tuberculosis of the spine, the mucopolysaccharidoses.

200 Accidental or non-accidental immersion of the child in an overhot bath.

201 (a) Supraventricular tachycardia.
(b) Wolff-Parkinson-White syndrome.

202 (a) Scalp skin defects.
(b) Patau's syndrome.
(c) The diagnosis may be confirmed by chromosomal analysis.

203 (a) A modified barium swallow.
(b) A flow of contrast medium into the trachea.
(c) H-type tracheo-oesophageal fistula.

204 (a) Rectal atresia. Impertorate anus.
(b) The marker is placed on the skin over the anal pit to give the investigator an idea of the length of the atretic segment.

205 (a) Prader-Willi syndrome.
(b) Chromosome analysis, which may show deletion of the short arm of chromosome 11 (p11-) in a minority of cases.

206 (a) Multiple dilated loops of bowel with no fluid levels.
(b) Meconium ileus, Hirschsprung's disease.

207 (a) Round face, hypertelorism, downward slanting eyes, and anteverted nares.
(b) Aarskog syndrome.

208 (a) Hydrocephalus and agenesis of the cerebellar vermix and part of the right cerebellar hemisphere.

INDEX

References are to page numbers